Don't Get Sick over Your Healthcare

Don't Get Sick over Your Healthcare

*Six Simple Steps to Take Control of
Your Healthcare for More Confidence,
Support, and a Healthier Future*

Dale White

Campbell Media, LLC

Don't Get Sick Over Your Healthcare

Dale White

Campbell Media, LLC
Published by Campbell Media, LLC

Copyright © 2018 by Dale White

All rights reserved.

Campbell Media, LLC
30767 Gateway Place, Suite 139.
Rancho Mission Viejo, CA 92694
Dale@preppedpatients.com

Publishing and editorial team:
Author Bridge Media, www.AuthorBridgeMedia.com
Project Manager and Editorial Director: Helen Chang
Editor: Jenny Shipley
Publishing Manager: Laurie Aranda
Publishing Assistant: Iris Sasing

Library of Congress Control Number: 2018903498

ISBN: 978-0-9997288-0-2 – softcopy
978-0-9997288-1-9 – hardcopy
978-0-9997288-2-6 – ebook

Ordering Information:
Quantity sales. Special discounts are available on quantity purchases by corporations, associations, and others. For details, contact the publisher at the address above.

Printed in the United States of America

DEDICATION

This book is dedicated to the three women who most profoundly shaped my life and world:

To my mother, who demonstrates unwavering strength, compassion, love, and humor in her everyday life.

To my daughter, the light that shines brightest for me and provides us all with hope that the future is in good hands.

And to Mary, who simply made the world a better place. Our eighteen years of marriage were too brief, but the time was filled with joy, adventure, and love.

ACKNOWLEDGMENTS

Much inspired the writing of this book. And similar to many life stories, this path was unexpected, with many twists and turns along the way. Not uncommon to those who have lost loved ones—through sudden events or a lengthy, painful illness—sorrow and helplessness are profound and lasting. Thankfully, human spirit is strong, and with help from family, friends, spirituality, and some truly random experiences, my daughter, Campbell, and I are again thriving.

One of the events on my journey which proved to be the most therapeutic was joining a healthcare organization, the last place many would have sought solace. My work in healthcare started with volunteering and developed into a career where my focus could shift to helping patients. As ten years rolled by, I knew the experiences learned in those multiple healthcare settings would also help patients. And here we are today.

My deep appreciation goes out to the dedicated doctors, nurses, clinic managers, and coworkers who taught me that nothing mattered more than caring well for patients. Thank you to the patients who challenged me and gave me a reason to get up and out of bed many days.

I owe a debt of gratitude to beta readers and advisors Ron White, Myra White, Campbell White, Heidi White, Marsi Gorman, Alex Vorobieff, Isaac Perez, Melissa Schenkelberg, the entire MLT team, and everyone else who convinced me this was a worthy project.

The team at Author Bridge Media is simply outstanding. A raw manuscript is truly just an idea. It takes sweat, talent, commitment, and gumption to convert that idea to a finished product. Thank you very much to Katherine, Julia, Jenny, Iris, Laurie, and Helen for guiding and reminding me that the result was well worth the effort.

CONTENTS

Part III: Maximize Your Care

Part IV: Follow Up

INTRODUCTION

An Increasingly Complicated System

Let's face it. Going to the doctor isn't anyone's idea of a fun time.

Why would it be? If you see the doctor because you're sick, you are already not at your best. And if it's a regular checkup, you're either anxious about something new being discovered or thinking, "If I'm not sick, what's the point?"

Even so, we all need to go to the doctor once in a while. And for most of us, the older we get, the more those doctor's visits will become a regular part of our schedule. This is just as true when we become parents or caretakers of our own parents or other elderly family members.

After all, our health and that of our nearest loved ones is one of our primary concerns in life—which is why trying to get the best possible care is often so confusing, frustrating, and downright intimidating.

In the past, if you started to feel like something was wrong, all it took was a quick phone call and you headed to the doctor's office. But now, scheduling a routine appointment can take weeks or longer.

Bottom line: there aren't enough doctors, appointment times, or staff to see all patients as soon as everyone—patients and medical personnel included—would like.

And once you finally get in to see your doctor (or, increasingly, a physician assistant), you have all manner of hurdles and challenges to deal with. Doctors are pressed for time, making it hard to get all your questions answered and medications explained and updated or to completely understand complex diagnoses or surgeries. And when we're under stress, worrying about our health, it's hard to even remember what we meant to ask in the first place.

Health-insurance policies are more complex than ever, offering less coverage for higher premiums. Unintentional billing errors are distressingly common—as high as 50 percent of all doctor's office billing, according to some experts. And many Americans aren't getting to the doctor as much as they need to, in part because there aren't enough medical transportation services available.

You can have all the tools in place for a quality healthcare experience: decent insurance, a good doctor, and even an appointment time you like. But it doesn't take much to throw a wrench into the works.

With all that, it's no wonder we hear so many healthcare horror stories from our friends, family members, and coworkers. We may have even experienced a few healthcare nightmares ourselves.

But does it have to be this way?

A Better Way to Get Better

The simple answer is no. No, it doesn't.

Healthcare is a complicated $3.2 trillion industry, but there is a way through the confusion and frustration inherent in such a system. What we need is something or someone to help each of us navigate the healthcare maze with knowledge and confidence.

In reading this book, you already hold the key to this mindset shift in your hands.

Armed with the practical knowhow, skills, and strategies I detail in the following pages, you'll become empowered to be more proactive with all aspects of your and your family's healthcare, resulting in better medical outcomes, health, and happiness for all those you hold dear.

The many benefits of taking this more proactive approach include the following:

- Being better prepared than ever for your doctor appointment, procedure, or surgery

- Feeling confident when speaking with your doctor and the clinical staff, and completely understanding all treatment options available to you

- Understanding the steps needed to reduce the chance of frustrating billing errors

- Saving time

- Saving money

- Reducing anxiety and frustration
- Developing a valuable relationship with a healthcare partner who will help you maximize your healthcare experience
- Having a better overall healthcare experience, which can lead to better overall health

We have an opportunity—perhaps even an obligation—to help ourselves and our loved ones successfully navigate the system.

No patient should *ever* be left behind.

A Life Interrupted

I didn't anticipate a career in healthcare.

For over a decade, I was fortunate enough to own and run a successful employment consulting company. Before that, I'd worked as a headhunter, where I learned that companies hire a lot of managers but don't select them particularly well. And once a manager is hired, few employers focus on retaining their best employees.

My consulting firm developed programs for companies that wanted to shift their staffing focus from hiring to selection and from managing people to keeping their best talent on the team. The positive changes we helped create for our clients made our work highly rewarding.

Then the unthinkable happened.

At the time, I had been happily married for fifteen years. My wife, Mary, was a personable, highly successful media business executive. We had an enthusiastic, thriving daughter, good jobs, and a solid family life—the American dream. But something else lurked uninvited into our lives.

Mary had been diagnosed with breast cancer more than ten years earlier. She bravely stared down the chemotherapy, reconstructive surgery, and stark reality and loneliness of the diagnosis back then, making the best use imaginable of her life—personally and professionally. Then, after years of remission, her disease made a sudden and dramatic return.

Again, Mary fought through more treatment options—some traditional and a handful of research studies. This time, however, the cancer spread rapidly. Mary's health deteriorated. She soon entered the palliative care phase and, eventually, hospice care.

We were navigating the unknown.

Every day, some new and daunting circumstance reared its head: new symptoms, the use of a different medicine. We needed home nursing for Mary, and we needed someone who knew the healthcare system well enough to take a more proactive approach to her care.

We needed help, and we needed it fast.

A New Path Forward

In the midst of this kind of crisis, it's easy to lose your sense of direction and begin to allow medical care to simply happen. The doctors advise you, but you don't know or understand what other options may be available. You're overwhelmed and bewildered, so the tendency is to simply trust and follow passively the first professional advice you receive.

The danger here is that less-informed, less-prepared patients often allow the *system* to make all of their treatment decisions. And while "one size fits all" can be a great approach when it comes to T-shirts, it fails when your health—or your life—is on the line. We can and should do better. That means becoming informed about all of our options and developing a new kind of relationship with our doctors to make sure these options are clearly explained.

What my family needed during my wife's illness was a healthcare partner who could guide us through all the complex and tricky pathways that stretched before us.

We were blessed to find that help in the form of my mother, Myra—a saint, if there ever was one. Having helped my dad through his decades of cardiac issues, she was an expert at navigating the system to get what they needed from it. And she was there to supervise everything as Mary, my daughter, and I struggled with the new reality we faced. Mom organized appointments, kept logs of notes after doctor visits, and helped maintain the needed medication schedule.

When we realized the medical options remaining to us were dwindling to nothing, the sense of helplessness I felt was unbearable. I had to do something—anything—to combat it.

My outlet was to volunteer at the large university teaching hospital in our town. I had no prior healthcare experience, but I ended up working four-hour shifts in the emergency room (ER). It was a Level 1 trauma center (the highest ER rating), often treating upwards of 200 patients daily.

If you're fortunate enough to have never spent time in an ER before, I can tell you this from personal experience: the amazing people who work there are committed to helping patients and their families, who often are facing their most urgent healthcare issue ever. These professionals work long hours under difficult conditions, but nothing matters more to them than helping sick patients.

A month into my eye-opening volunteer experience, I was approached by an ER supervisor who asked me why I was there. She told me I wasn't a typical volunteer, and she'd noticed the way I enthusiastically interacted with patients, their families, and the ER staff. I filled her in on what was happening in my personal life and told her that somehow being in a healthcare setting and helping others gave me strength during my wife's final months.

"Well, maybe you've found your calling," she said. "You should consider working here instead of volunteering."

My immediate reply was polite dismissal. But as I went on to work my volunteer shift, I couldn't help but wonder: What *would* it be like to work at the hospital full time? I had to admit it was appealing: more of the joy of helping people in times of dire need, more of the adrenaline rush of the ER's crazy pace. Wow, I thought. Where was this coming from? I was a successful business owner, after all. What a crazy idea to give all that up!

A month later, I was hired in that same ER.

Your Guide to Navigating the Maze

In most cases, the person in my position was the first contact a patient had with the ER. I checked in patients and provided any support needed by the ER department's nursing staff, doctors, medical residents, pharmacists, and social workers.

At the time, it didn't matter to me that this was far less financially lucrative employment. I closed the consulting company I'd operated for fifteen years, understanding that this was the start of a new and more fulfilling career.

For the first time in a long time, I was in love with my work. It was intensely stimulating to work in that environment. And helping patients and their families, along with hospital staff and my coworkers, was extremely challenging, but equally rewarding.

While my parents were living with us and helping care for Mary, my father suffered a stroke. He didn't recover, and weeks later, we lost him. Mary passed away shortly thereafter. I'd worked in the ER for just over two years when I knew it was time to take a break.

Knowing I wanted to remain in healthcare, I shifted to the same medical school's clinic operations when I resumed working in the fall. My title was float receptionist, and, instead of checking in patients at one location, I now worked in *twenty different clinics*, all with different specialties, including orthopedics, ophthalmology, cardiology, dermatology, neurology, psychiatry, and many more. Every day was different, and I was fortunate to be working with world-class physicians and talented clinical staff.

The patients I encountered in my new line of work had a lot in common. They sought great healthcare and were generally optimistic. But I also saw in them something more intimately familiar. As I had been during our family's health crisis, most of these patients and their families were primarily *reacting* to the healthcare system around them, rather than being proactive in their approach.

Mostly, they seemed to drift through the system. I noticed early and often that the patients who best managed their healthcare were treated more quickly and seemed to have better results.

The skills I'd developed as a business owner and employment consultant were useful in the healthcare industry, too. I saw the big picture for patients, but realized that—through no fault of their own—many were unable to successfully navigate or utilize the medical-care process.

Back when I started my healthcare employment, I couldn't have envisioned creating a patient-care handbook. But the more experience I gained, the more I came to realize that many people could benefit from what I had learned.

That's why I wrote this book—for you. Whether you're currently a patient yourself, a caretaker of a friend or loved one who is ill, or just someone who wants to learn to better understand and navigate our challenging healthcare system, I know you'll find much useful information in the following pages.

How to Get the Most Out of This Book

The information in this book has been organized into four parts:

- Tools for Healthcare Success
- Understand the System
- Maximize Your Care
- Follow Up

Each part contains vital information you'll need to manage the healthcare system successfully.

I recommend you read through this book once, marking up the pages when you encounter bits you find to be particularly useful or applicable to you and your circumstances. Then, after you've read the book once, read it again. As when you watch an entertaining movie for the second time, you'll see what you missed the first time and learn even more.

Not everything in the book will apply to you, but a great deal of it will. You can take as much or as little as you need from it, but do yourself a favor and try to incorporate at least three of these new ideas into your healthcare routine. Just three. And once you have those mastered, add three more.

Either way, you'll still need to go to the doctor, and you'll still face the challenges of navigating the healthcare industry. Since this is a reality all of us face, it's better to prepare yourself. Someday you may find that your life—or the life of someone you hold most dear—may literally depend on your healthcare knowledge and preparation.

As may be obvious from the lack of extra letters after my name, I am not a medical doctor. The only person any of us should trust with medical answers is a medical doctor—not me, or even a nurse, and certainly not the insurance company.

So if this book leaves you with any questions about pursuing medical care, don't hesitate to take action. Call your doctor or another doctor's office for medical treatment. Never wait. Delaying making an appointment or putting off your healthcare in any way is never a good idea. No matter your financial or personal situation, if you think you need to see a doctor, you're right. And you need to do it now.

The Knowledge and Confidence You Need to Thrive

Over the last ten years, I've helped 50,000 patients just before and after their healthcare appointments. In that time, I've borne witness to the fear, confusion, frustration, intimidation, and disappointment in their eyes, or in the eyes of their loved ones, as they struggle to navigate a confusing system in a time of need and anxiety. The drama of an ER visit or a surgical procedure multiplies those feelings several times over.

Everything else aside, I wrote this book for you, *the patient*, and for those of you who want to help your loved ones, friends, and others get the best medical care possible.

This journey we will take together will hopefully be more than just eye-opening for you and for those you're helping. We'll go far beyond the anticipated challenges of having a productive appointment. I'll offer real-world examples of how to turn your experience from one you may dread to one you embrace as an opportunity to get the optimal diagnosis and treatment from your doctor visit.

I can picture you entering the clinic, the ER, or the hospital with confidence. You may not feel your best physically—after all, you're seeing the doctor. But one thing you won't have to worry about is drifting through the experience unaware and unprepared.

You'll be empowered.

You will gladly schedule that appointment. And you'll know how to get your doctor to explain what the diagnosis means, your treatment options/program, and the follow-up plan so that you fully understand each crucial piece of your care.

The staff will notice your preparation, your confidence, and your upbeat attitude. These will result in more attention and a more focused appointment, meaning you'll get better healthcare. And better healthcare promotes improved health and happiness—not just for you, but for those who love you as well.

The concepts I'll be introducing are simple things you can incorporate into your healthcare regimen with astoundingly powerful results. Some of these are rooted in common sense, and some may require a shift in mindset—but all will benefit you, your loved ones, and anyone you are helping to manage healthcare for—both now and in the long run.

Are you ready to take the reins of your healthcare experience? We have a lot of road to cover.

Let's get started!

Part I

Tools for Healthcare Success

INTRODUCTION TO PART I

From Anxiety to Empowerment

One of the biggest hurdles many of us face when we get sick is the feeling of helplessness and frustration that results when we perceive a lack of control about what's happening to us, as well as *when* and *how* we receive care. Often, we feel 100 percent at the mercy of the appointment scheduler, our insurance company, the clinic, the staff, the pharmacy, and the doctor. Worse, the shortage of doctors creates a situation where we feel even less in control.

We fear we're going to be told what to do and when to do it, with little or no input as to what we feel is best.

But there are *always* other options available to you as the patient. You just have to know when, where, and how to look for alternatives. You also need the confidence it takes to speak up, ask for what you need, and keep advocating for yourself until you get it.

Since confidence requires knowledge and preparation, the first thing you'll need to navigate the system successfully is a better understanding about how it works in the first place. Your newfound confidence in your own abilities will then help you steer your own course through whatever medical challenges come your way, rather than feeling as though all you can do is follow a prescribed course of treatment in which you have no say.

Here in part 1, we'll answer questions like these:

- What are the most important things I should consider when trying to navigate the healthcare system?

- Who can help me stay on track and manage my healthcare goals?

- How can I help my family members or other loved ones manage their healthcare needs?

- How can I better hear my doctor's diagnosis and understand my treatment plan?

- How do I remember all that my doctor told me in the short few minutes we spend together?

With the tools and techniques that you're about to learn at your fingertips, you'll rest easier knowing that the next time you walk into a doctor's office, you're going to feel empowered to get the best possible healthcare for yourself, your loved ones, or anyone else you're there to support.

Chapter 1

Building Blocks to Healthcare Success

A New Approach to Our Healthcare

We rightfully respect and sometimes even have a little hero worship toward our doctors. For those of us who've experienced medical hardships and have seen firsthand what a difference doctors make in providing care, treatment, and improved quality of life, this is only natural. When we have a doctor we know and trust, we tend to feel confident he or she is providing excellent diagnoses and medical-care treatment plans.

But even so, we should never feel herded into or out of the office. We cannot be rushed. We have a right to the appointment date and time that fits our schedule best. We have a right to expect that the doctor will make time for our questions—because we're not leaving the exam room until we understand the diagnosis and our treatment plan going forward.

Yes, in adopting this approach, we are going somewhat against the traditional medical-care grain. But we're doing it with a positive, friendly, and confident attitude—and that makes all the difference.

In this chapter, you'll learn six key techniques for getting the very best out of your healthcare experience.

Your Six Building Blocks to Healthcare Success

This industry has taught me much about patients and their families, doctors, medical staff, and insurance providers and how each group is dependent on each other.

Through my experience, I've determined there are six basic, rock-solid fundamentals to ensuring the best available healthcare. Faithfully practicing these components will allow you to most effectively manage your doctor's appointments and, ultimately, your entire healthcare process. These fundamental steps, in order, are as follows:

1. Identify your healthcare partner (HCP) and communicate this person's role to your doctor's office. This person will help you navigate the complexities of the healthcare system by going to your appointments with you (when needed) and helping you stay organized and on top of things.

2. Prepare for every appointment in advance by:

   ♦ confirming your appointment date, time, and location

- always carrying your updated insurance and medication cards

- having your health questions ready for the doctor and his or her staff.

3. Don't leave the appointment until you are confident you know and have repeated back to the doctor the treatment and follow-up plan. Always schedule your follow-up appointment *before* you leave the doctor's office.

4. Develop an intimate relationship with your health-insurance coverage.

5. Create a contact list to identify who at the doctor's office can help you the most.

6. Accept and plan for the fact that your appointment, surgery, procedure, testing, hospital stay, or any other medical-care experience will likely not go exactly according to plan and will almost always take longer than you expect.

And we're going to do all of the above with an upbeat, positive attitude. Really?

Yes, really!

Some people reading this book are going to believe I lean toward supporting physicians over patients. Others will feel I'm giving patients the confidence to make unrealistic demands of their healthcare providers. And still more may say the insurance industry is behind this work.

My only goal, though, is to help you, the patient, or your children, parents, grandparents, friends, and even coworkers to navigate this challenging, complex world of healthcare. I'm sharing ten years of my experience observing what patients do well and what they can improve. And I can say with confidence that, if you follow the six steps I've outlined above, you will drastically improve your odds of receiving excellent medical care and patient service.

This really works. I see many patients from all walks of life struggling with all manner of medical challenges every day. And, as I've said before, the ones who consistently see the best outcomes within the system are those who manage their care using these building blocks for success.

You'll see me refer back to these core principles throughout the rest of the book as I break down each step in greater detail. First up is establishing the best secret weapon you'll ever have at your side in this journey: your designated healthcare partner.

Chapter 2

Identify Your Healthcare Partner

A Patient's Story

A friend once asked me what sort of equipment we had at the hospital that completely erased all memory of the time between entering the emergency room and just before leaving the hospital. He was joking, of course, but his comment points out something that many patients have experienced— lost time when recovering from a serious injury or illness during hospitalization.

One day he wasn't feeling well and noticed some of his facial muscles weren't working normally. When he told his wife, she immediately drove him to the ER. An experience with her mother a few years back suggested that her husband might be experiencing stroke symptoms. She didn't tell her husband her fears, but she knew time was a huge factor, and when she relayed the information to the ER check-in desk, her husband was roomed immediately.

The doctors soon confirmed her intuition was correct: her husband had suffered a mild stroke. My friend remembers only getting to the ER. After that, it's all a blur.

Thankfully, he was admitted to the hospital, went through a battery of tests, received a consultation, and was given medicine and a treatment plan. The entire process took three days, but he remembers little of this time. He just remembers hearing the initial news that he'd suffered a stroke.

But his wife was there, and her quick action and careful note-taking during his treatment made all the difference in his care and recovery. That's the value of having a thoroughly experienced and knowledgeable healthcare partner.

Circumnavigating "Fight or Flight"

You may have heard of the "fight or flight" response common to all animal species, including humans. Our highly adapted adrenal system grants us enhanced perception, strength, and stamina in the middle of a crisis, allowing us to survive dangerous scenarios that would otherwise likely get us killed. Even so, our adrenal system can also make us a liability to ourselves when it comes to getting the medical treatment we need in the wake of such circumstances.

The same stress response that allows a 130-pound mother to singlehandedly lift a car off her child after an accident can also cause mental confusion, disorientation, and even memory loss while under duress. Since this coping mechanism is hardwired into us, we need to learn to work around it and make sure we receive the care we need when we're under stress.

This is why it's so important to have a designated HCP like my friend's wife in the story above. It's also why, when an ER doctor has important news or a clinic physician needs to communicate a treatment plan to a patient with a brand-new diagnosis, he or she always asks if someone else is there with the patient to receive the information.

That concerned friend or relative is much more likely than a rattled patient to retain and immediately process important information. The HCP is also much more likely to ask questions specific to the patient's medical history and lifestyle, bringing up important considerations that might otherwise be overlooked.

At the end of the day, having an HCP to advocate for us is one of our most powerful keys to healthcare success. Your HCP is someone who can help remind you of what was discussed or any instructions given at the appointment and the plan moving forward.

Having an HCP is just plain good preventive medicine, similar to having a personal fitness trainer or a gym workout partner—someone who can remind you of the big picture and hold you accountable.

In this chapter, you'll learn the amazing benefits of designating an HCP to help you manage your health more efficiently and proactively. We'll cover whom you should ask for help and how to approach that person. Let's get started.

Who Needs a Healthcare Partner?

You may be reading this and thinking that I'm referring only to elderly patients, those with disabilities, or special-needs patients. This is a common misperception.

The truth is, we all would benefit from having a healthcare partner.

Mothers and fathers of younger children know this. They're already the HCP and advocate for their children.

There are many more compelling reasons why each of us needs someone else to help look out for our health. I'll go through some of these below.

They Remind Us of Things We May Have Forgotten to Mention

When you're able to thoroughly answer questions about your health, your healthcare providers can do the most for you as a patient. Some patients prefer to say less about their health; they don't want to be a bother. But your doctor needs to know everything about your health history. With your HCP at your side at an appointment, you'll be more likely to answer medical questions completely. As needed, your HCP can help remind you to fill in any medical-history gaps.

They Keep Us Calm—or, at Least, Calmer

Our perception of what constitutes calm, appropriate, and pleasant behavior or demeanor and the doctor's perception of these things may differ quite a bit. You've been waiting what seems like an awfully long time for your appointment, and you're concerned about your health. You may also be in pain or discomfort, so you're a little amped up emotionally. Having someone you know and trust by your side can help you keep a level head, which will lead to a better experience and clearer communication between you and your provider.

They Make Us Feel More Confident

We gain confidence with the doctor and other clinical staff when our HCP is with us. We're also much more likely to ask questions. This is human nature; there's strength and confidence in numbers.

That said, having your HCP with you is not a license to run roughshod over your healthcare providers. The best way to continue getting great healthcare and patient service is to keep all parts of the medical-care process working in your favor. Doing this with confidence *and* with a pleasant attitude will always get you further, faster.

They Help Us Better Understand Diagnoses and Treatment Plans

Even if we're paying close attention to what the doctor says, sometimes there's a disconnect between what was said and what we actually heard. Having another (calmer) set of ears and eyes in the room can help make sure we're really on the same page with the doctor. If we don't understand something important, our HCP may be able to explain it in terms that make more sense than the doctor's explanation.

They Can Help You Follow Up

You may find that, after your appointment, you're unsure of some of your treatment plan details and need to ask some questions. (When do I start taking the medication? What else am I supposed to do?) If you're like most people, you might feel embarrassed or uncomfortable calling the office to ask these kinds of things. For some, this discomfort can lead to *never* calling to get the needed clarification, and either winging it or skipping the treatment plan altogether, and that can be truly detrimental to good health.

Your HCP is a perfect person to make that phone call on your behalf if you need a little help with this. Please know that as someone who has worked in a variety of doctors' offices, I appreciate patients and their HCPs who call back with clarification questions after appointments. This shows you care and that you understand how important the treatment plan is.

Whom Should I Pick as My Healthcare Partner?

Let's talk about who qualifies to be your HCP. As you might guess, this person can be anyone you know and trust to help you, or maybe someone you don't know that well but who is trained to do the job. There's a good chance that someone from the following list would make an excellent HCP:

- **Your spouse or life partner**: For many people, this seems an obvious choice. No one knows you better, and this person is probably able to get you to the doctor when you hesitate to go on your own. (Men, I'm in this boat with you.) One of you is probably more organized, so that partner should keep records of appointments, file your appointment summary forms (more on these coming up soon), and stay on top of insurance. Men, this doesn't mean you can automatically just hand this off to your partner. It's incumbent on each of us to step up and be a true HCP to our partners.

- **Your parents**: No one cares more about you than your parents. In my line of work, I consistently see patients' parents as the most concerned and protective HCPs. Emotions can run high with these partners—after all, no matter how old you get, you're still their baby! But typically, a mother or a father will do anything for you. The older generation is also typically well educated in the healthcare arena. Heck, my mom could have written at least half of this book.

- **Your grandparents**: Who knows more about the healthcare system than your grandparents? They've seen it all and are a wealth of information. They will make you feel confident and truly care about your health. Even if they aren't your healthcare partner, ask them for advice. They have a lifetime of valuable experience.

- **Your child**: As mentioned, there's a real opportunity to introduce or build on your children's healthcare education. They can learn from your experience and help themselves—and others—as a result. It will take work to get them involved if they're young. But your children will have a life partner someday, and possibly children of their own. Help them to help you, and they'll be miles ahead of their contemporaries.

- **Another family member**: I've often made the mistake of asking a patient if the person with him or her at an appointment is a spouse or partner. Many times, it's a sister or brother. You'd think I would learn! But blood is thicker than water, and your sibling, niece or nephew, uncle or aunt, or anyone else in your family qualifies as an excellent HCP.

- **A friend or coworker**: Promise to return the favor and you are already helping create an HCP network. Your friend has heard your stories and knows much about your health issues. He or she knows your preferences and lifestyle and, especially if close to your age, relates well to you. After all, most of us spend more time with our coworkers at work than with our life partners!

- **A neighbor:** This depends on the nature of your relationship. If it's just a person living next door, you might not feel comfortable sharing your health history with your neighbor. If you're friendly, though, perhaps you would be comfortable asking a neighbor. Since they live close, neighbors are a natural choice for getting you to and from your appointments. And they'll no doubt appreciate you returning the favor if they need help in the future.

- **A volunteer:** Some volunteer agencies (often found through your church or one nearby) are large enough to offer patient transportation and health-advocate volunteers. Search online for a local organization that offers patient services. Call a large local church. Ask at a larger healthcare clinic or hospital. University teaching hospitals are likewise a great source of volunteer options.

- **Someone you hire to help you**: Professional healthcare advocates are also available to you. Not just a caregiver, the health-educated partner provides advice on important health decisions and can arrange transportation, confirm appointments, and follow up with your doctor and medical staff. This can be expensive, but it's an option with growing popularity.

Once you've decided who your HCP is, always sign the "consent to verbal communication" paperwork available at your doctor's office or pharmacy or through your insurance provider. List your HCP by name and include his or her contact information, if requested, on this form. Every doctor's office has these forms.

If you don't make these changes to your paperwork, then due to privacy laws, the doctor's office, insurance company, or pharmacy might refuse to communicate with anyone other than you regarding your healthcare. Bigger healthcare operators follow this law to the letter. Even if you did everything else right, forgetting to notify your doctor or clinic about your HCP will complicate the process.

Ask about this form, and update it at your next appointment.

Asking Someone to Be Your Healthcare Partner

Some HCPs are obvious choices for you, but others are not so obvious. In any case, you'll need to ask one of them to join your healthcare team. But you also don't want to scare that person off with fear of a long-term commitment. Here's a sample script for how I would approach this conversation:

"I'm very committed to managing my healthcare, and I have things in order for now.

I could use someone, though, to help me do this better.

I need a healthcare partner who will know my health history, medications, and health needs.

I trust you and appreciate the way you manage your own healthcare.

Would you mind if I discuss with you the process I'm going through, and would you be comfortable helping me stay on top of my healthcare?

I don't want to scare you off thinking this is a major commitment, but I will be more than happy to do the same for you."

At first, this conversation may not be easy for you. As I mentioned earlier, many of us want to take care of ourselves. We are mostly private about our personal needs. We don't want to bother others with our medical issues, especially if we seem healthy and capable of managing them on our own. And everyone else is busy, right?

This kind of thinking is missing the point.

Much of our society is reaching an age where more healthcare will be necessary. We need to help each other if we're going to get the appointments we want and the face-to-face time with the doctors we need and—most importantly—to understand the treatment and follow-up care plan.

Practice asking someone to join your healthcare team. It will likely make someone feel great that you trusted him or her enough to ask.

And yes, you can have more than one HCP. In fact, you *should*. This will increase the chances of having someone available when you need the help. Just remember to give back as well. If you receive help, give back twice as much. If you have one healthcare partner, offer your services to two others.

The Most Important Advocate for Your Health . . . Is You!

Ultimately, each of us must be our own best healthcare advocate. From time to time, situations will prevent your regular HCP from being with you at an appointment or during a hospital stay. Think of your HCPs as fellow advocates on your team. But *you* are your healthcare manager.

Next up, I'll cover some of the finer points of being a healthcare partner for someone else. Once you're able to provide this assistance for someone in your life, you'll gain increasing confidence in managing your own healthcare experience.

Chapter 3

How to Be an Amazing Healthcare Partner

Partners in Health

As a healthcare partner, you've volunteered yourself to assist a patient in navigating the complexities of the healthcare process and possibly also driven the patient to and from appointments or procedures when needed. Few people offer as much of themselves as you have in stepping up to be someone's HCP. On behalf of patients, clinic staff, insurance providers, and doctors everywhere, I thank you.

Know that your role as healthcare partner is a vital one. Sometimes you will need to step up and take the reins in the process, but there's a fine line between being a partner and being a director.

Since you cannot possibly attend every single appointment, perhaps the single most important thing you can do as a healthcare partner is to teach your patient partner how to be his or her own best healthcare advocate. You can do this by viewing each appointment as a teaching opportunity.

When you share what you've learned about how to navigate the system effectively—from this book, other trusted resources, and your own experience and history—you're empowering your patient partner to have more agency in his or her own care. The more your patient partner learns, the more effectively he or she will be able to self-manage and take charge, whether you're there with that person or not. What's more, that patient will be able to teach others from experience, helping even more people to achieve the confidence and knowledge needed to obtain the best care.

On the other hand, if you fail to teach your patient partner what you know about the process and how to maximize his or her care, you'll be setting the patient up to overly rely on your assistance. Remember, it's important for patients to have the confidence, knowledge, and tools to be their own best healthcare advocates.

If it helps, you can think of your patient partner as the captain and yourself as his or her copilot. This is a journey you'll take together, but the patient partner is in the driver's seat. You're there to make sure he or she does not take a hasty wrong turn in a moment of stress or fatigue.

In this chapter, I'll outline the key points of how to be an effective healthcare partner, including tips and advice for what to go over with your patient partner before an appointment and how to best help that person maximize care.

Healthcare Partnering 101

First off, as a healthcare partner, you'll need to be prepared to assist your patient partner with any (and possibly all) of the following tasks:

- Confirming the appointment for the patient with the clinic

- Arranging transportation as needed

- Assisting the patient in communicating with the clinic staff and the doctor

- Helping the patient summarize his or her medical diagnosis and treatment plan at the doctor's office by completing the appointment summary form either during or immediately after the appointment

- Scheduling the patient's follow-up appointment before you leave the doctor's office

Remember that as an HCP, you're a significant part of the process. The assistance you are providing is vital. Just knowing that someone else is there for support can alleviate a lot of the stress and anxiety patients feel when dealing with not feeling well and navigating the system to receive the diagnosis and treatment needed to get better. And having a second set of eyes and ears in the exam room can make all the difference in making sure that we are communicating clearly with the doctor and other key medical staff.

Now that you know what to expect, let's move on to how to prepare before going to an appointment with your patient partner.

What You Need to Know

Before you go to a medical appointment with your patient partner, there are some things you'll need to discuss first. That way, you'll be prepared to effectively help the patient to manage his or her own care.

To this end, make sure to talk to your patient partner about the following topics *before* the appointment:

- The patient's health history
- Current medications (also ask for copies of the patient's health-insurance cards)
- Problems the patient has had with medications or past procedures
- The health concerns to be addressed with the doctor during the appointment
- The patient's healthcare preferences: how he or she wants to interact with the doctor
- What you should do if the patient is too sick to communicate or becomes incapacitated

- Does the patient have an advanced care directive or healthcare power of attorney prepared?

- Which family members should help make decisions for the patient, and how can you contact them?

- The patient's appointment date, time, and location

Being prepared ahead of time will clear the way for a productive, efficient appointment, allowing you to do your best to assist your patient partner in getting the best possible care.

Final Thoughts on Being a Great HCP

The best HCPs are prepared, organized, informed, and compassionate.

They prepare in advance, familiarizing themselves with the patient's health history, medications, and concerns. They're organized enough to stay on top of key details such as the time, expected length, date, and location of appointments, as well as the mode of transportation and any related needs. They stay informed, turning to the patient for updates on recent changes in health or medication and new symptoms or troubling side effects. And they exude compassion by boosting the patient's confidence, listening empathetically, and striving for patience when needed.

Combined, these qualities help to create excellent doctor appointments, resulting in your patient partner receiving better care and having better overall health. I know, because I've seen this to be true time and time again.

Another important tip I can offer you as a new HCP is to please be respectful to everyone at the doctor's office, especially the patient you're helping. Occasionally, I see an HCP who is overbearing. Please remember that, as a healthcare partner, you are just that: a partner. You add true value to the doctor's appointment experience by working with the patient and healthcare providers to make sure the patient receives the care he or she needs.

There are times when frustration with your patient partner may occur, especially if he or she is running late or isn't completely prepared for the appointment. Some patients—both young and old—move slower or faster or think differently than others. Frustration can easily build, especially with family members. When you need to, take a deep breath and remember the bigger picture of what you're here to do.

Also keep in mind that doctors and their staff perceive patients based on previous appointments. You are part of this patient's healthcare team now, so your demeanor and behavior will impact how the patient is perceived. As the HCP, you have a great opportunity to set an upbeat tone for the encounter. Try starting things off by introducing yourself to the person at the reception desk and saying something like,

"I'm here to assist my friend and to help you and the doctor, so please let me know how I can make your job easier."

Helping someone navigate the complex healthcare process isn't easy and can come with its fair share of frustrations, but it is also incredibly rewarding. People talk about giving their time and energy to important causes to make a difference. We tend to think more globally, leaning toward larger charitable groups, church programs, or political organizations. This is all worthwhile work, but as an HCP, you'll be making a big difference one-on-one for someone you know in a way that is deeply personal.

That's an incredible gift. And you'll certainly appreciate having someone else return the favor for you if and when you need it.

Now that you know the ins and outs of how to be an effective healthcare partner, I'll share with you another key tool I've developed for getting the best out of the system. Next up: the appointment summary form.

Chapter 4

The Appointment Summary Form

The Smart Approach to Your Healthcare

One challenge many of us face when at the doctor's office is trying to remember everything the doctor tells us in the brief time we have together. This is often compounded by stress about our health or simply not feeling well, along with all the other thoughts and concerns that may be running through our minds.

Still, it's important to find a way to recall what the doctor tells us so we can be sure to consider and incorporate suggestions, understand our diagnosis, and follow through on our end with our treatment plan. For most of us, our memories are less than perfect, so one great way to make sure we remember key pieces of information given by the doctor is to record them using a standardized form that we bring to the appointment.

I call this the appointment summary (AS) form. I created it as a tool for you, the patient, and your healthcare partner (HCP) to help you do the one thing most patients could do better: prepare for your doctor appointment. There's nothing complicated about this form. It's easy and simple to complete. And once you're armed with it, you'll feel confident, empowered, and ready to see your doctor.

With the AS form in hand, you can not only record and track the information you get from your doctor at each appointment, but also remind yourself to bring up all of your current symptoms, medications, and concerns. Having all of this written down spares you the anxiety and trouble of trying to remember it, giving you greater confidence and the best chance of attaining a quick diagnosis and treatment plan.

If you don't use a tool like this, you put yourself at risk of forgetting to bring up key pieces of information your doctor needs to treat you effectively or letting important pieces of your overall medical-treatment puzzle fall through the cracks.

By using this form, you're making a big statement to your doctor and his or her staff. The medical team will appreciate that you're respectful of your appointment and their time. You cared enough to prepare, and it shows. Even though filling in the blanks with your doctor present may feel intimidating, you'll show them you mean business. And it's entirely possible your doctor will give you a few more moments of undivided attention as a result.

In this chapter, I'll teach you how to use this incredibly useful tool to manage your healthcare more efficiently and proactively.

Appointment Summary Form

Patient Name:	**Medical Assistant:**	**Phone Number:**

Doctor: **Specialty:**

Appointment Date/Time: **Confirmed: Y/N**   **Location:**

Healthcare Partner: **Transportation:**

Purpose of Appointment - My Health Concern:

Questions for the Doctor/RN:

1.

2.

3.

Appointment Results:

1. Diagnosis:

2. New medication/update to current medication:

3. Treatment Plan:

Follow-Up Plan & Next Appointment:

1.

2.

Using the Appointment Summary Form

On the previous page, you'll find a blank copy of the AS form. Take a moment to familiarize yourself with each section.

For the best results, fill out the first six boxes *before* your appointment and the last two either during or immediately after. In particular, pay attention to the sections titled "purpose of appointment" and "questions for the doctor/RN." Jotting down your notes and questions here before the fact will help you communicate more clearly with everyone at the doctor's office, from the receptionist to the doctor and everyone you encounter in between.

On the next page, you'll find a sample completed healthcare form. You can download all of the forms in this book at my website, http://www.preppedpatients.com/

On the site, you'll also find information useful to maintaining your healthcare-management fitness. Do your family and friends a favor by referring them to the site. Please share it with anyone you know who might benefit from the information and tools available there.

Appointment Summary Form

Patient Name:	Medical Assistant:	Phone Number:
John Doe	*Jane Smith*	*123-456-7890*

Doctor:	Specialty:
Dr. Carter	*Orthopedic*

Appointment Date/Time:	Confirmed: Y/N	Location:
Friday, June 20, 2018 - 2:00 p.m.	*Yes*	*North Clinic - 4th Floor*

Healthcare Partner:	Transportation:
Richard	*Richard*

Purpose of Appointment - My Health Concern:

Right wrist pain for 2 weeks

Questions for the Doctor/RN:

1. What are possible causes of the pain?   *Overuse/sprain*

2. Is it serious? Is it treatable?   *Not serious; rest will keep 3. it from becoming chronic. Very treatable.*

3. How long will it take for my wrist to heal?   *6-12 weeks of rest/treatment*

Appointment Results:

1. Diagnosis: *Sprained wrist/ligament*

2. New medication/update to current medication: *Increase ibuprofen dosage*

3. Treatment Plan: *Get an X-ray, discuss results. Use ice/heat 4 times per day. Discuss possible physical therapy.*

Follow-Up Plan & Next Appointment:

1. *Discuss X-ray results with RN in 2 days*

2. *Follow-up appointment - Tuesday, August 6, at 10:30 a.m. - South Clinic 1st FloorDr. says to cancel follow-up appointment if symptoms disappear, tell the RN if cancelling*

Notice that in the "questions for the doctor" section, the patient or Richard—the patient's HCP—has included the answers provided by the doctor during the appointment to the questions that the patient entered on the form prior to the appointment.

By using the form, the patient has in one handy place all the basic information needed regarding the injury and how best to complete his or her course of care.

I want to share a few additional tips regarding the AS form.

First, don't feel constrained by its format. If you don't have enough room to fill in your answers, flip the page over and use the open space on the back.

Second, one of the most important things you and your HCP will do during an appointment is to read back your notes to the doctor and be sure you understand the treatment plan moving forward. The time to do this is *during the appointment.* Communicating with the doctor (or nurse practitioner or physician assistant) afterward is rarely as effective as doing so face-to-face during your actual appointment. It's also more difficult and time-consuming to verify this information after the fact, so be sure to do it while you're still talking in person.

Some doctors or staff at larger medical practices will see you taking notes at an appointment and offer to give you an "after-visit summary" report before you leave the office. While these summaries are helpful, the office-generated report often doesn't include a complete description of your appointment and will likely not show the specific questions you asked. Writing your own answers in your own words on the AS form, even if it takes a few moments, is more beneficial, because only then can you make sure *all* of the key information you need from your doctor has been covered and thoroughly explained.

I suggest keeping a file or binder for storing these forms once they've been completed so you have them in one place and can refer back over your healthcare history as needed. You can even put a more sophisticated system together, filing the forms by doctor specialty or type of procedure (i.e., lab work, surgery, etc.). Your past completed forms also make an excellent resource for sharing your health history with a new doctor or with your family or HCP.

Here in part 1, you've learned the building blocks of success for getting the most out of the healthcare system, as well as the tremendous benefits of having an HCP by your side. Next, we're ready to move on to part 2, "Understand the System." In this portion of the book, we'll dig into the "meat and potatoes" of the healthcare system, including how to work with and choose a doctor and how to prepare for your appointment.

Part II

Understand the System

INTRODUCTION TO PART II

Forearmed for Success

Patients visit doctors for a variety of reasons, including regular checkups, urgent conditions, help with a variety of physical and emotional issues, and surgery. People arrive at their appointments with different levels of preparedness, but I've seen, time and time again, that those who come best prepared can expect to see better overall healthcare outcomes.

Since being prepared for your medical appointment, procedure, or treatment requires an understanding of how to take advantage of everything the healthcare system has to offer, we first need to understand the system. Only then can we successfully find and navigate the best pathway to improved health and happiness.

The danger of not being prepared is that the healthcare system will be glad to direct us if we allow this, rather than the other way around. There's a world of difference between passively hoping it all works out and taking the reins to do your best to ensure a positive outcome. The chief benefit of being a prepared patient is being well equipped to get the needed medical care that leads to healing and a healthier, happier life.

Here in part 2, I'm going to give you the information you need to be prepared, as well as an inside look at how medical clinics work. I'll also share some easy-to-implement tips on how to best use the system. I want to help you learn what I've learned firsthand as a medical front-desk employee.

We'll cover several topics, including:

- What do you need to better understand your doctor, and how will that help you get better care?

- What happens behind the scenes at a medical practice?

- How does the staff function and think?

- Who can help me navigate the healthcare maze the most, along with when and how?

- Is there someone who can explain my insurance and help with a billing problem?

- How do I get the appointment that best fits my schedule?

I'll help you answer all of these questions and more, while sharing a few real-world examples along the way. Most important, part 2 will give you solid, concrete examples of steps to take to keep you on top of your healthcare game.

Once you understand the system better and can prepare yourself to use it to its full advantage, you'll develop the increased comfort and confidence you need to be an active participant in making decisions for your own health. Let's get started!

Chapter 5

Understand Your Doctor

The Power to Heal

Doctors are my heroes. I admit it: I'm in awe of what they can do.

For ten years, I've witnessed doctors handle countless medical emergencies with a calm, yet deliberate, and experienced approach. I've watched patients who had no pulse brought back to life and drug overdose victims survive near-death experiences.

I've seen pediatric physicians reassure new parents that their infant would survive and thrive after a complex heart or brain surgery. I've looked on as ophthalmological surgeons provided light, color, and even sight to patients who never believed they'd have it again. And I've experienced the amazing, sincere kindness demonstrated by doctors helping patients through the final stages of their lives.

Doctors and the work they do are certainly special, but at the end of the day, they're human beings just like you and me. With all the incredible things they do for us, it can be easy to think of them as superheroes, but it's important to realize they *don't* actually have superpowers. And since doctors are not mind readers, they need to know how you feel in order to do their jobs effectively. This means you need to respect both their and your own time by being prepared for your appointment and communicating your concerns clearly.

The benefit of communicating effectively with your doctor is a better working relationship with him or her. Over time, your doctor will come to appreciate the fact that you share the information he or she needs to keep you healthy. This improved trust and communication directly results in better healthcare outcomes for you, the patient. The risk of not communicating effectively is that if the doctor doesn't have all the necessary information, he or she can't make the best decisions for your care. As a result, you could end up with the wrong diagnosis, medication, or treatment—leading to everything from wasted time and increased frustration or suffering to serious medical complications, or worse.

Our lives are *literally* on the line here. It's up to us and our HCPs to update our doctors on our medical condition at each visit, tell them which medications are and are not working, and share our hopes and concerns for treatment and a return to better health.

In this chapter, I'll cover what you need to know to better understand your doctor so that you can communicate effectively and get the care you need to live a healthier, happier life.

The Doctor Next Door

The first and most important thing to understand about doctors is, as I said above, that while their ability to save lives sometimes makes them seem like superheroes, they are every bit as human as the rest of us.

This also means that, like anyone else, each doctor has a specific personality, communication style, and management style.

Some doctors are more friendly than others. Some spend more time with you during your appointment than others. Some, in fact, are more competent than others, in which case they may believe they don't need to spend as much time with patients individually in order to provide the best quality care. And some of them are even correct about this.

Because I have split my time between more than twenty clinics in my healthcare employment, I've worked with doctors with work styles that range all over the spectrum—both pleasant and not so pleasant. Regardless of personality type or demeanor, all of the doctors I've worked with have one thing in common: at the top of their list of professional goals is genuinely wanting the best for their patients. At times, this fact can get lost from the patient's perspective due to personality differences or what is sometimes perceived as brusqueness on the part of the doctor.

As an example, I once had an elderly patient who showed up at the last second before the clinic was about to close for the day and needed a special medication filled right away. This required a signature from a doctor, but I knew that this particular doctor was often quick to make a getaway as soon as the last patient was out the door and was probably already headed out.

I approached the medical assistant (MA) and pleaded the patient's story. To the MA's credit, she chased the doctor into the parking lot, stood in front of him, and held out the prescription. He was on his cell phone, shook his head, and got into his car.

Not the result we'd hoped for!

I understood the situation. Like most doctors, this one was incredibly busy, juggling multiple responsibilities and demands, but I knew the patient would be disappointed, and I dreaded telling her she wouldn't be able to get the medication that day. As I approached her and her husband, my front-desk phone beeped. It was the doctor calling from his car. A minute later, we had the signed prescription.

In my experience, doctors are like good parents in that they are mindful of their responsibility to those they provide care for. Most are consistently appreciative and respectful. They understand that mistakes are going to happen, and they work incredibly hard to make sure they're doing right by each and every patient.

Get the Best Out of Your Doctor Experience

While medical and clinic support staff are needed to make what doctors do possible in the first place, doctors themselves remain the heart of our healthcare team. Nothing and no one replaces them and what they do for us as patients. No matter whom you see at the doctor's office, the physician is ultimately responsible for your care.

During an appointment or a consult for most nonurgent medical issues, the doctor will look over the patient, ask questions, maybe run a few tests, and then typically present the diagnosis and map out a treatment plan.

One thing to keep in mind to help manage your expectations about seeing your doctor is the fact that there are not enough doctors to go around. This is a prevalent problem all over the nation, and, because of it, many doctors maintain an overly ambitious appointment schedule. This means they are often running behind schedule—sometimes frustratingly so.

Remember that one of our building blocks for healthcare success is to understand that an appointment, a procedure, or our estimated recovery time after a procedure is almost always going to take longer than expected. To minimize any inconvenience to your schedule, always estimate that more time will be needed than you think for a doctor appointment.

And know that nothing replaces face-to-face time with your doctor, so when you need this, *say so.*

Once you better understand how to communicate effectively with your doctor, you'll be better prepared to discuss key information regarding your health, which will lead to better outcomes for you as a patient. Next up, we'll learn about the other professionals who work with doctors at the clinic and how they can help us along our healthcare journey.

Chapter 6

Who Else Is on Your Healthcare Team?

Get to Know Your Service Providers

Without question, the team at your doctor's office is determined to provide their patients with excellent care. But who are these folks exactly, and what is each person responsible for? If you don't know this information, how will you know where to go when you need help with a specific question or problem related to your care?

That's just it. You won't.

Part of being a well-prepared patient is knowing whom to go to at the doctor's office for specific questions related to your treatment, billing, insurance, or any other concerns that may come up. That's because knowing who's who will allow you to direct your questions to the appropriate staff member. Understanding the role of each member of the medical team will help you to better navigate the healthcare system.

If you don't understand the specific roles and jobs of the employees at the doctor's office, you may end up wasting both their and your own time asking the wrong questions of the wrong people. This, at best, can lead to frustration on both parts. Worse, it can negatively impact your relationship with your healthcare providers and the level of care you receive.

On the other hand, knowing whom to go to for specific information streamlines your healthcare experience, reducing frustration and ensuring you get the information you need *when* you need it. After all, you have only a limited amount of time allotted to you during your appointment, so knowing the roles of team members will save both you and them valuable time that can then be better spent addressing your particular concerns.

This level of added preparation will also help you differentiate yourself (or your patient, if you're a healthcare provider) from the patients who *don't* take the time to educate themselves about what each person at the doctor's office can be expected to know or be responsible for. As a result, you'll get more time, better answers, and, as a result, a better healthcare experience.

In this chapter, we'll cover who's who at the doctor's office, the increasing role physician assistants and nurse practitioners play in our care, and other important players like your pharmacy staff and insurance provider.

Once you know your healthcare team, you'll be equipped with the knowhow needed to get the best service and care from each person you come across in the healthcare system.

First, let's look at who works at your doctor's office besides the doctor.

Who's Who at the Doctor's Office

Depending on the size of the practice—running the gamut from small, private clinics to offices that are part of a larger healthcare network system—a variety of personnel, each with specialized knowledge, skill sets, and expertise, can help you make the most of your healthcare experience.

Below, I'll break down who's who at the clinic so you know what to expect when communicating with medical employees and providers, and how best they can assist you.

Receptionist/Front Desk

This person is the face of the clinic and the first person you come in contact with when you arrive for your appointment. This person is also typically responsible for answering the phone, so be patient if you get an "I'll be right with you." If you have a good first experience, it's likely because the front-desk team is friendly, helpful, compassionate, and efficient.

The duties of the front-desk team include:

- checking you in for your appointment
- verifying your personal information and insurance, asking you to sign paperwork, and collecting your co-pay

- communicating any urgent issues to the nursing staff or doctor
- scheduling follow-up appointments

They can help you by:

- keeping you updated on how long your wait time is for your appointment
- finding a follow-up appointment time that best fits your schedule
- helping connect you to the billing department if, for example, you have a billing problem from a previous visit

A handy tip: Keep in mind that *you* also make a first impression on this important team member. If you're pleasant, polite, ready with your information, and appreciative of their help, you'll help free them up to focus on how best they can serve you.

Nurse/Medical Assistant

This is the person who will take you back to the exam room. Many practices have a nurse—an RN, LPN, LVN—on staff. But it's a common trend for the doctor to use an MA or technician for the exam room check-in. These professionals are trained and certified, but they don't have the same level of education as a licensed nurse. Their experience in the position may be even greater than a nurse's, however, so don't discount their ability. Their responsibility is to "set the table" for your doctor by:

- verifying your medications
- checking your vitals
- asking about any medical-history changes
- discussing the purpose of the appointment

They can help you by:

- being a sounding board for any other medical conditions you may want to address with the doctor in addition to the primary reason for your visit. This person can help you decide if you need to discuss it that day or if you should schedule another appointment.

- helping you schedule upcoming lab work, tests, or procedures based on your availability. The doctor won't have time to go through those details with you, so that's this technician's job.

- talking with the receptionist on your behalf if you need to make a series of appointments. "The doctor says to work her into his schedule" goes a lot further from this staff member than coming from you.

A useful tip: Don't assume this encounter is just the warmup to seeing the doctor. The information the nurse or MA records will go straight to your chart and is one of the first things the doctor sees in the exam room. The doctor may not know why you're at the appointment, but the notes entered by the MA or nurse are vital in providing that information. Be aware that it's common—but not guaranteed—that the exam room check-in details will be discussed with the doctor by the medical-team member before the doctor enters the room.

Billing Coordinator/Insurance Expert

This person is responsible for the payment side of your visit, an often overlooked (by the patient), but vitally important, part of your medical-care experience.

It's important to note that it's cost effective for many physicians to contract out their billing service, which explains why many errors might occur. In this case, it's yet another set of people handling the billing process. This also means they don't know the patients and may not yet be completely familiar with the doctor's practice. They deal only with billing and procedure codes, names, addresses, insurance providers, and other details.

Take a look at any bill from your doctor's office. If there's an outside billing agency, you'll see a different address and contact phone number listed somewhere with a "billing phone" or "billing address" section. If it's a phone number different than your doctor's office, that's the one to call to make sure you're speaking with the person who can actually assist you.

The billing coordinator handles:

- verifying insurance and confirming active coverage. I can't tell you how many times a patient's insurance is active one day and then suddenly inactive. There are myriad reasons why this can happen, so you need this person on your side to determine the cause. He or she can usually check your coverage in real time, instantly.

- obtaining authorizations for procedures (i.e., radiology, biopsies, surgery).

- educating you about your insurance coverage.

- acting as your billing advocate with insurance providers if you don't understand your bill or if there's an error.

- giving you highly accurate estimates of co-pays due and out-of-pocket expenses for procedures, tests, and more.

When a billing error occurs, it's often due to patient insurance information not being updated, incorrect information in your account, or the possibility of human error or oversight. Your policy identification numbers are usually complex, so they're easy to enter incorrectly. If you're up to speed on your insurance coverage, benefits, out-of-pocket expenses, and deductibles, you'll at least know what's coming after an appointment or surgery. A strong knowledge in this area may even allow you to confidently negotiate amounts you owe.

Clinic Manager/Office Manager

This is a mostly administrative position, responsible for overseeing the staff and interacting directly with the doctors regarding certain patient, insurance, and business decisions. You probably won't come in contact with this person regularly. He or she is, however, another potentially important ally.

As the person closest to the doctor's "peer" on the staff, the clinic manager can get the doctor's attention and discuss concerns you may have about your care or that of a family member. The manager also serves as the contact person if you're not making progress with the doctor. For instance, the clinic manager may be able to convince the doctor to open his or her schedule later on Thursdays to see after-school patients or to speak more directly with you during and after your actual appointment.

The clinic manager is the only staff member I've seen who can comfortably call the doctor by first name. That means something.

Conversely, the clinic or office manager can easily tell you "no" if you're trying to negotiate a discounted or cash price because you're uninsured or want to pay less than your co-insurance deductible. In my experience, the doctor is *always* the best person to speak to when negotiating price.

Tip: Always get a name and contact information for each key person at the doctor's office, including the clinic manager. These are the people who can help improve your patient health experience. On your side, they are always valuable allies.

Seeing a Physician Assistant (PA) or Nurse Practitioner (NP)

Here's a big trend in the healthcare industry: when it comes to seeing your primary care provider, you are increasingly likely to see someone other than your doctor at your office appointment. Today, in many larger medical practices, your appointment is likely to be with a nurse practitioner (NP) or a physician assistant (PA) up to 30 percent of the time. Over the next ten years, that percentage is estimated to increase to upward of 50 percent.

We're looking at a worsening national shortage of primary care physicians: by 2025 we will be up to *twenty thousand* shy of the number we actually need. Due to the aging of our population base, the use of the NP/PA has become an absolute necessity.

In addition to being a scheduling godsend for healthcare providers and patients alike, the NP/PA is generally well regarded on both sides of the industry. In my experience, these practitioners are highly approachable and helpful. While they work with and are supervised by doctors, they aren't as bogged down with the administrative weight of the healthcare business, as most doctors tend to be. So NPs and PAs are not only highly educated and competent (both generally have a master's degree or the experiential equivalent, and both are licensed and certified nationally and by their state), but also typically able to see you more quickly and to create more time for you during your appointment than the doctor can.

To share a brief anecdote, a friend, concerned about the possibility of appendicitis in his daughter, recently took her to a busy emergency room for abdominal pain and fever. The person who organized and directed all of their care for this visit was an NP. Not once did a doctor enter the room, though I'm certain the NP consulted with an ER physician, as is the protocol. It turned out this was a case of the flu, but the examination, lab work, treatment plan, and prescription were all developed and delivered by the NP. The process went smoothly, and my friend's daughter recovered using the prescribed course of treatment.

The increased availability of NPs and PAs is a great benefit for practices—and for patients—that utilize them. An appointment with your primary care doctor that couldn't be scheduled for days or weeks could, with these practitioners, be scheduled for just a few days away—or even the same day.

Keep in mind that since they are increasingly used to fill in for doctors, an NP or PA, rather than your doctor, may be the one to see you when you get to a regular follow-up, postsurgical, or even an urgent-scheduled appointment. Many of us assume we're seeing our regular doctor, and we may not remember if we were told we may see an NP, PA, or another practitioner. This isn't an intentionally deceptive move by your doctor's office; rather, it's often standard practice now, partly out of necessity so that you can be seen more quickly rather than having to wait days or weeks for your appointment.

However, as vital a role as NPs and PAs play, it's also important to keep in mind that they are not medical doctors.

As always, *you* are your own best healthcare advocate. If there's a realistic reason for concern in dealing with anyone other than the doctor, you should feel empowered to speak up. (You don't want a PA alone diagnosing and treating your cardiac issue or diabetes, as an example.) If you're even slightly unsure about whether you're seeing a practitioner different from your primary care provider, ask the scheduler or receptionist for their input. That way you can ensure everyone is on the same page about the best choice of provider for you.

An important tip: If you've been assigned to an NP, PA, or someone else and haven't seen your doctor in three office visits, insist that you see your doctor at your next appointment. Chances are if you've been seeing another clinical staff member, your health is pretty good. That's great news! Just don't allow your doctor to become a stranger.

Other Key Healthcare Team Members

In addition to the helpful folks who work at your local clinic, there are other people you'll encounter when navigating the healthcare system. You'll especially want to concern yourself with your pharmacy staff and your health-insurance provider.

At the Pharmacy

The pharmacy is staffed primarily with pharmacy technicians. Large pharmacies process hundreds of new and refill medication prescriptions every day. But thanks to automated prescription-filling equipment, safety checks, and experience, the pharmacy gets the prescription filled correctly more than 99 percent of the time.

Developing a positive relationship with your pharmacy and the people who work there can save you money and time. Your local pharmacy tech can help you by:

- updating your insurance coverage, contacting you when a prescription is ready for refill and pickup, and advising you on medication choices, both over-the-counter and prescription.

- helping you access coupons that may reduce your prescription cost. Next time you're at the counter, ask if there are any current coupons that will help you save on your order.

- signing you up (often for free) for services like a prescription-drug savings card, which can benefit patients with no insurance or those with less-than-desirable prescription coverage.

- asking your doctor for a less expensive option for your medication, such as a generic brand or a similar (but different) medication. I've seen patients save up to 90 percent of what they'd normally pay thanks to this kind of assistance!

At Your Insurance Provider

Although they might sometimes feel like opponents, insurance providers are an important part of your team. Developing a relationship with your insurance provider is vital. We'll talk more about managing your insurance in later chapters, but as with other key healthcare team members, always work to identify a reliable, competent, go-to contact at the insurance company. This will save you a world of time and hassle.

Chapter 7

Choose Your Doctor

The Right Doctor, the Right Care

There will come a time when, even if you're happy with your current doctor, he or she will retire, or you'll move, or your insurance will change and no longer consider your healthcare provider as "in network." Alternately, you may experience changing health conditions that require you to see a new specialist.

Since our lives can literally rest in our doctor's hands, and each of us is bound to be faced with the need to pick a new doctor at some point, it's important that we are prepared to make an informed decision.

I sometimes see prospective new patients come in and ask whether the doctor has frequent openings in his or her schedule or works out of a specific office—entirely ignoring the doctor's length of experience, reputation for being patient-friendly, or receptiveness to patient questions. This is risky, because having a doctor who can see you more often, but with whom you can't communicate effectively, is not going to result in the kind of care you're looking for.

Why does this matter so much?

When you think about it, we invest a lot of time in choosing a new car or a place to live. That's because we know these decisions will affect us every day—potentially for a long period of time. We want to feel good about choices we make to improve the quality of our everyday lives. Taking the time to choose a doctor who's right for you is much the same.

You are much more likely to schedule—and keep—your healthcare appointments if you have a solid relationship with your doctor and care team. It just makes sense. Conversely, if you're dreading telling your doctor that your treatment plan didn't work or that you have a new medical concern, you might see your doctor less frequently or be more inclined to let those first smaller symptoms turn into something bigger.

Aside from your preferences for doctor-patient communication styles, medical competency should be your biggest concern and the reason you take your time in selecting a doctor. Investing some time in research—whether it's asking other doctors or friends and family or checking state and other physician-reporting websites—will pay off by matching you up with a better doctor who will help you attain better healthcare results. I've seen surgeons with no bedside manner perform medical miracles. Some doctors have absolutely no interest in hearing your opinion, but they are superb technicians who know their trade. Ultimately, you need to determine the combination of personality and competency you prefer and, maybe more important, the combination you can live with.

The overall benefit of doing your research and selecting a doctor who is right for you is experiencing better healthcare outcomes that result in a healthier and happier life for you, the patient.

Of course, if you're in a health maintenance organization (HMO) plan and need to see a specialist, you'll have to go through your primary care doctor before being referred to the specialist. (If you go straight to the specialist, you risk being stuck bearing the entire cost of the bill. Yikes!) Even so, you can use the tips in this chapter to verify that the specialist you've been referred to is not only covered by your insurance but also actually the doctor you *want* to see.

In this chapter, I'll cover what to consider when choosing a new doctor to ensure you select the right physician for you, as well as how to streamline your search to save time and effort. I'll also teach you a useful tip to help you avoid any nasty surprise costs after you've had your first visit with a new doctor.

Let's dive in!

The Technician versus the Active Listener and Consultative Doctor

Doctor work styles are as different as our personal styles. Some are friendly, some less so. Some are more focused on the science of what they do, and others try to focus equally on the science and on the people they actually serve—or what many refer to as bedside manner.

If you're committed to being an active manager of your own care, one type of doctor to beware of is the kind that practices a "technician" work style. These doctors are often wonderful scientists, able to pore over patient data and quickly reach scientific conclusions about the best treatment plan. But they're also more likely to tell you what to do based on what they see empirically, rather than taking your input under serious consideration.

"Trust me," they'll say, "this is the best way to proceed with your care." This type may even view your HCP, with AS form in hand, as a schedule destroyer. When being treated by a technician-style doctor, patients may find they leave their appointments confused, not entirely sure of what was discussed or the plan going forward.

If you're more comfortable with this type of doctor, be prepared to voice your input. Insist on full explanations of your diagnosis and treatment options, and make sure you understand the game plan for your treatment moving forward. Your HCP and the AS form are both fantastic tools available to you for these purposes.

At the other end of the spectrum, there are the less technical, more methodical, but still highly competent doctors who will want to know much more about your concerns, your health history, and maybe even your treatment preferences.

This type of doctor is much more likely to embrace the idea of you having an HCP in the room to help guide you to the best possible care. I refer to these providers as the active-listener-and-consultative doctors.

Some patients will gladly spend an extra hour, if needed, waiting for doctors with this active-listener-and-consultative work style to finish with other patients. Other patients find this type's less-assertive (compared to the technician style), "we should give this a try" approach to be an uncomfortable fit.

The active-listening doctor is going to be different in many ways. First, he or she will actually look at you. These days, you'll notice that doctors and their medical teams spend a lot of exam-room time looking at and entering data into a computer screen. In the "old days," doctors took physical notes and stored that information in a paper medical chart for future reference. Today, your medical record is usually stored in a computer database. The doctor wants to input information during your appointment, so his or her eyes and attention go to the computer screen.

This consultative listening physician, however, is more likely to look at you and confirm what you've said before turning to the computer. Some doctors can expertly do both tasks—active listening and inputting data into the computer—simultaneously, similar to how someone giving a speech does so while reading from a teleprompter, but doesn't make this completely obvious.

This doctor will appreciate and embrace the idea of you having a completed AS form when you walk into your appointment. He or she will most often ask, "Do you have any other questions we should address?" The technician-type of doctor, on the other hand, is less likely to ask the same question.

It's also more common for the active-listening doctor (or the medical team) to follow up with you after your appointment, testing, procedure, or surgery.

These are only two examples of doctor-patient interaction styles. There are others. Some doctors are more paternalistic, not just listening but also directing your care and often making medical choices for you. These doctors will say they're disappointed you didn't follow their treatment plan to the letter. This doctor-patient style is better for patients who want direction and are less interested in making their own healthcare decisions.

Another doctor-patient approach growing in popularity involves a doctor who offers an opinion on your medical condition and treatment, asks for your input, and then leaves the room to "huddle" or consult with a medical team. Upon reaching a conclusion, the doctor returns to the exam room to share a concrete treatment plan with the patient. Many patients feel good about this style because their opinion was factored into the final treatment recommendation.

Let me be clear that both the technician and the consultative listener have strengths. Mostly, we are talking about a difference in the style of patient interactions. Doctors from both styles are likely highly competent, experienced, and effective. But the perception of which approach is *more* effective or simply more comfortable will differ from patient to patient and may be heavily influenced by the doctor's interactive tendencies.

Here's how I view my choices. If I'm choosing a primary care physician (PCP), I want a doctor who spends time with me and addresses all of my health concerns in a caring, compassionate way. I'm happy to spend more time at those appointments because this type of doctor takes a holistic view of my health issues.

For a knee surgery with an orthopedic specialist, however, I'm less concerned with wanting this kind of approach. In that sort of situation, my preference is more focused on "let's get the knee repair completed and do it quickly and efficiently so you can send me on my way to start my rehabilitation." Alternately, if I'm looking at facing a long battle with cancer, I want my oncologist to be more of a listener and consultative provider.

You will know what feels best for you under different medical circumstances. The important thing is to be aware of these different doctor-patient work styles so that you're better armed to ask for and receive exactly the type of care you want and need.

Streamline Your Search

Once you've taken work style into consideration, how do you actually choose the best doctor for your medical-care needs?

First, understand that this discussion isn't about which doctor styles are *better* than others. Rather, it's more about developing an awareness of what's best for you as a patient, considering your own medical needs, communication style, and other preferences.

The worst way to pick a doctor is to choose a random name from a list. On the other hand, you don't want to spend hours and hours on this decision. To streamline your search and save time, ask for referrals from people you know and trust.

First, ask for recommendations from family members, coworkers, or other healthcare navigators. There's no better way to find out how a doctor performs than from someone who has been a patient. You can ask about the doctor's patient-communication style, his or her ability to stay on time with appointments, and even about the efficiency and friendliness of the staff.

Another person you might not think to ask is your current doctor. Doctors often refer their friends and family to their most trusted colleagues, and you can ask for the same recommendation with a quick call to the office. As in our examples above, tell the doctor you appreciate a considerate doctor who is willing to spend time with you and listen to your input, but that you're looking for the right blend of someone who's a strong technician *and* is patient-friendly. Your doctor will understand what you mean.

A question that always works for me when I'm asking for a referral from doctors I already know is this: "If you were selecting a new doctor for this issue, whom would you recommend to one of your family members?"

The next step, once you have the names of some recommended doctors, is to check to see if they're covered "in-network" through your insurance. In most cases, you can do this quickly online. You'll double-check (and triple-check) that this information from your insurance plan's website is current and accurate later on—we'll get to that—but for now, just check the website.

Once you've verified that a recommended doctor is in-network, online reviews can help you further narrow your search. That said, you may want to toss out the very best and very worst reviews and focus on the general comments. In any case, you'll learn a lot from these sites, but it's best to combine the information you find here with your referrals, using the reviews to confirm or contrast what you learn from your friend, family member, or other personal contacts.

That way, you get a bigger piece of the overall picture.

Double- and Triple-Check That the New Doctor and His or Her Specialty Is Covered

Once you find a doctor who comes highly recommended, is in-network, and has good online reviews, it's time to take the next step: double- and triple-check that they're in your insurance network and that the service or specialty you plan to see them for is also covered.

Wait a second. Didn't we already do this?

Yes, in part. But as I mentioned in the last section, it's important to check and recheck insurance requirements because this information can change practically overnight. The next step is to call your insurance provider to verify that your potential new doctor is definitely in the network and that the cost of your appointment will be at least mostly covered. (Ask specifically how much the out-of-pocket cost will be so there are no surprises.) More important, make sure that the doctor in question is covered in-network *for the specific specialty or service you plan to see them for* (i.e., OB GYN, internal medicine, cardiology, psychiatry, etc.). Some doctors have multiple specialties, and the last thing you want is to go in assuming your appointment is covered because the doctor is in-network, and then find out the specialty or service you saw the doctor for isn't covered.

A lot of people skip this step and then wonder why that first doctor's visit winds up with a much bigger price tag than expected. Worse, once a problem or misunderstanding like this has occurred, it takes *much* longer to sort it all out on the phone, which can be incredibly frustrating. And chances are, even after all that, you'll still end up footing a bill you weren't expecting.

Do yourself a favor: call. It will take only a few minutes, and it can save a lot of time, headaches, and money later on.

Once you've verified all of this information with your insurer, the last step is to actually call the doctor's office and speak with a scheduler or another front-office worker, such as the receptionist. This call has two purposes:

- To ask if the doctor is accepting new patients
- To verify *on the office's end* that the doctor accepts your insurance coverage

Be very specific about your insurance coverage, and have your insurance card ready so you can provide any information the medical staff needs.

If everything checks out and you've made your decision, great! Go ahead and make your appointment while you have the scheduler on the phone.

On the subject of scheduling your appointment, next up we'll look at some tips and tricks for just that.

Chapter 8

Schedule Your Preferred Appointment

Speak Up

As we've discussed, one of the chief responsibilities of the receptionist at your clinic is to schedule patient appointments. Those of us in this role use expensive software platforms to help us get the job done, but our most valuable resource for this duty is *you*, the patient. So if you don't seize the opportunity to tell us what you need, chances are you're going to get the first option that pops up on our computer screen, rather than an appointment that actually works well for you.

Since it means you'll be in a better mindset and a better position to receive optimal care, getting the appointment time that best fits your schedule leads to better healthcare outcomes. If you have to take time away from work during the middle of the day or at a time that's similarly inconvenient in your schedule, you'll be watching the clock more closely and will have less attention and focus for getting the most out of your appointment. Similarly, if you're in a rush, you may not want to take time to ask the important questions you need answered during your examination.

The same applies if you're an HCP. Your family member or friend will benefit from your full attention and focus on making sure that both patient and doctor have all the information they need to make good decisions and follow through on the chosen treatment plan.

In this chapter, we'll cover the ins and outs of how to get an appointment time that best fits your schedule, including my insider tips for how to communicate better and more effectively with your scheduler.

The Lay of the Land

Before you schedule your appointment, it's important to have a full picture of how scheduling works. As we've covered, there is a significant shortage of doctors in our country compared to the patient population.

That means that if you urgently need an appointment and are trying to be seen as soon as possible, this is going to be difficult to manage from the outset. It's particularly hard to get a same-day appointment because your doctor's schedule is already full—maybe even overbooked. Even so, if your medical issue is urgent, most physicians will work to fit you in.

This will, however, require flexibility on your part. If the staff says the doctor can see you at 10:30 a.m. today, then you need to make yourself available for that time slot. You might also need to be open to seeing a PA or NP if your doctor is not available.

I'm in your corner. I know you're not feeling well, and you might have to struggle to get transportation on short notice. But your scheduler is doing the best he or she can to get you the care you need as soon as possible, often under difficult circumstances on the clinic's end. So it's important that you're willing to meet the scheduler halfway.

Primary care visits, tests, radiology, and lab appointments are relatively easy to schedule, while more complicated procedures like surgeries or other in-patient hospital services tend to be much less flexible when it comes to scheduling.

Get the Best Appointment Time

When it comes time to schedule an appointment, first determine what the ideal appointment time is for you. Some of this is based on your general availability or preferences. For instance, many retired patients tend to prefer late-morning or early-afternoon doctor visits, while parents with school-age children want those late-afternoon/early-evening appointments.

Below are some techniques you can use to help land your preferred appointment:

- **Be pleasant.** You may have noticed that being courteous is a recurring theme in this book. If you think you're being pleasant enough, turn it up another notch and smile (even over the phone, people can *hear* a smile). Try saying something like, "I know you're busy, so thank you in advance for helping me find a good appointment time. I appreciate it."

- **Have your calendar ready, and tell the scheduler what day and time works best for you.** Otherwise, you'll end up with the first day and time that pops up on their screen or the best time for the doctor.

- **Take your time.** Don't let the scheduler rush you, but remember that your scheduler has other patients to assist, so be ready to pick an appointment in a reasonable amount of time.

- **If you don't get the appointment you prefer, ask to be put on a cancellation list.** Most doctors' offices have one. If not, you can reasonably call once a week to see if there's a cancellation at a time that works better for you.

- **Get on a first-name basis with the receptionist/ scheduler.** Again, having a go-to contact person at the clinic will help you get the best from your experience. If the scheduler knows who you are and remembers your friendly, appreciative attitude, he or she may just call you if that coveted appointment time you want becomes available.

- **Schedule your follow-up or next regular appointment before you leave the doctor's office.** The best time to schedule any appointment is *now* versus later. The further in advance you schedule, the better chance you have of landing an appointment that fits your needs and preferences.

Chapter 9

Prepare for Your
Doctor Visit

Your Healthcare Motto: Be Prepared

By now, you've carefully selected your doctor, and you have your preferred appointment scheduled. Way to go!

Now you're ready to prepare for your appointment. This is an important step, but it's one that many patients skip. This extra effort, however will significantly increase the quality of your appointment. Since our health hangs in the balance when it comes to getting the most out of our medical appointments, it's vital that we prepare ourselves in advance for a smooth, efficient doctor's visit.

There are many reasons why it's important to be well prepared for your appointment. Just as an attorney prepares final arguments for a trial or a politician practices a campaign speech, there's something delightfully comforting about knowing you're ready to see the doctor even before you walk through the doors of the clinic. You'll be confident, you'll feel a little more relaxed, and the staff will notice.

That all works to your benefit, because it helps you project a positive, pleasant image of yourself to the staff, which in turn makes them more eager to help you get exactly what you need out of your appointment.

What's more, once you've done your prep work up front, you can focus on truly hearing what the doctor and the staff have to say. And if they don't cover the issues you know you need to discuss, you can easily refer to your AS form for a quick reminder.

If you skip preparing, however, you'll find that you tend to simply "flow through" the healthcare system rather than act as a good healthcare advocate for yourself. After all, if you're taking the time to go to the appointment in the first place, you might as well prepare yourself for success.

In this chapter, I'll teach you what steps to observe before your appointment to make sure things go smoothly. You'll save yourself an incredible amount of time and frustration and set yourself up for a lifetime of successful navigation of the system.

Before Your Appointment

Before you're seen by your doctor, be sure to observe the following important steps to ensure you're prepared for maximum success when the actual day rolls around.

Confirm Your Appointment

Even if you think you have the correct date and time down, call or email the office one week before your actual appointment to verify. If you call a week ahead and there's a problem (i.e., your appointment has mysteriously been cancelled or was never confirmed to begin with), you can plead with the staff to try to work you into the schedule.

You'd be amazed at how many people stumble over this seemingly simple issue. The reality is that many forces and distractions compete for our time and attention every day, which can easily lead to human error when we jot down our appointment information. And yes, the appointment scheduler may have made an error, too. It's especially important to confirm your appointment if you don't receive a reminder phone call, text message, or email from the office at least a few days in advance. That's a red flag for sure!

Verify the Clinic Has Your Current Contact Information

Making sure your contact information is up to date at the doctor's office is another important way to avoid unforeseen problems. Doctors' schedules change frequently, and if we can't reach the patient, we leave a message and ask for a return phone call. This means, however, that we rely on you, the patient, to make sure to tell us if and when this information has changed.

When you call to confirm your appointment—and each time you visit the office—verify with the receptionist that they have your correct phone number(s), email address, and emergency contact listed, as well as permission to communicate with your emergency contact as needed.

Confirm Your Transportation and/or Healthcare Partner's Availability

Contact your HCP well in advance of your appointment to inquire about or confirm his or her availability to go with you. If you'll need assistance with transportation to and from your appointment, make sure to make arrangements in advance so that when the day comes you don't have to worry about being late or missing your appointment.

Carry Your Health-Related Cards

Always carry your insurance and medication cards with you so that you have them when you need them. And make sure they're up to date! It's also a good idea to keep extra copies of your cards with your important papers at home, in your car's glove compartment, or even as digital images on your phone.

Complete the First Part of the AS Form

As we've discussed, one of the best tools available to you before, during, and after your appointment is the appointment summary form. Before your appointment, write down the important details of when and where your appointment is, along with which doctor you're seeing. Also include the reason for your visit (i.e., symptoms, name of doctor who referred you, etc.) and any questions you want to ask the doctor. It's unbelievable what a difference it makes to have this information written down and with you.

Also be sure to keep your half-filled-out form in your purse, wallet, or car so that the form will be close by when you need it. That way you can't possibly forget to bring it to the appointment.

Prepare a List of All Current Medications and Supplements

This is a big one! There are a host of reasons the doctor wants to see this list, including potential problematic medication interactions, dosages that require adjusting, a newer or less-expensive medication that might work better for you than your existing medication, and many others.

Be sure to list any medications you're allergic to, as this can literally save your life in some cases. Be sure to update your medication and supplements list regularly between doctor's visits, and keep it handy as part of your health records—perhaps in the same place you keep your past AS forms. And if you're currently *not* taking any medications or supplements, that's just as important for your doctor to know.

Know Your Medical History

When it comes to your health, you are your own best historian. Knowing your medical history (and making sure your HCP knows it, too) empowers you to communicate effectively and efficiently with your doctor and other healthcare providers to get the care you need as quickly as possible. Write your health history down and keep it with your other important healthcare paperwork. Schedule reminders using your calendar to update this history every six months.

Request Medical Records from Other Doctors in Advance

When you schedule an appointment with a new doctor, ask the scheduler if the office will need your previous medical records. If the answer is yes, contact your previous doctor as soon as possible to get this process started, since it can take some time. As a patient, you have the right—typically free of charge—to have your previous medical records sent to your new doctor electronically from your primary care provider and any specialists you may have seen.

Assume Your Appointment Will Take Longer than Expected

Remember our healthcare success building blocks? This is one of them. You can spare yourself the inconvenience and hassle of running late back to work or other appointments if you realistically anticipate that your appointment will likely run long.

Appointment times can vary depending on appointment type. An annual physical examination can typically take up to an hour, although if you're seeing a new doctor, your first visit will always take longer. Other procedures, like a quick blood-pressure check with your existing primary care provider, should take just minutes. Bottom line: the best times to ask about appointment duration are when you schedule and then again when you confirm the appointment.

Chapter 10

Communication Is Key

Every Parent's Nightmare

The ER where I worked was located in a town with a large university. Not surprisingly, the local college students occasionally partied a little too hard. After too many parties, these students, suffering from dehydration and abdominal pain, sometimes needed to come to the ER for help. They weren't seriously ill, but they certainly felt as though they were!

Sometimes, after these kids were admitted for treatment, their parents would call long distance and ask to speak with their child. Due to national patient privacy laws, however, if a patient is over the age of eighteen, hospitals need permission from the patient to even *confirm* he or she is at the ER—even to immediate family members. And it was common for students in this position to refuse permission, perhaps out of embarrassment or just to avoid a confrontation.

This created a great deal of anxiety and frustration on the part of those parents. You can perhaps imagine some of the things my coworkers and I heard from them on the phone.

We sympathized, of course, but that's the law. And even at our clinics, parents can be surprised when we direct our attention to their child once they turn eighteen. We advise the new adult to include their parents, if they're comfortable doing so, in all "consent to communicate" paperwork. Still, the new adults have a right to refuse.

The moral to this story? If there are people in your life that you wish to keep in the communication loop between you and your doctor's office, it's vitally important to communicate this to your doctor's staff.

Understanding Patient Privacy

Healthcare privacy laws are strict. And fines for healthcare providers are significant if they are caught violating privacy or HIPAA (Health Insurance Portability and Accountability Act of 1996) laws. There is flexibility for doctors to discuss *some* medically necessary information with family members or caregivers, but only if the patient doesn't object. There are exceptions for patients who are nonresponsive or critically ill. But for healthcare workers, a single violation of these policies is often met with immediate suspension, or even termination.

Since maximizing our healthcare experience means working with friends and family—including our HCP—to manage our health, it's important to make sure these people have access to information about our care from our doctor's office. This means ensuring you have filled out and returned to your doctor's office any necessary paperwork needed to verify who is and isn't allowed access to such information.

Making sure you have this paperwork filed in advance means you're covered and prepared to receive the best possible care, whether you're in for a routine appointment or faced with an unforeseen emergency. In either case, you'll want your HCP and any other designated emergency contacts to have access to your doctor and his or her staff.

When you take care of this paperwork proactively, you will save precious time and eliminate red-tape complications for your HCP and family. Give your HCP and a reliable family member a copy of any form that gives permission for your doctor to communicate with your HCP and that same family member. That way, they have proof they're allowed to be kept in the loop when it's needed.

The last thing you want is to be put in a situation where your HCP or one of your close loved ones—like your spouse, parent, or adult child—urgently needs information about your health from a doctor or a hospital and is unable to access it, or even to find out if you're all right after a sudden illness or accident. In this case, these people will not be able to confirm your appointment times, treatment plans, medication refills, or even that you've been seen by one of the doctors at the facility in question. All of the above represent what's at stake if you don't communicate with your doctor's office and get your paperwork in order.

In this chapter, I'll cover the two main forms of patient privacy paperwork you need to consider to be fully prepared for any future healthcare needs: consent to communicate paperwork and the advance healthcare directive. Once you understand the purpose of each of these forms, you'll be able to confidently complete them. Then you can relax, knowing your healthcare bases are covered, no matter what life has in store.

"Consent to Verbal Communication" Form

This form is always available from your doctor at any appointment. It may also be part of the new-patient paperwork you complete at your first appointment with a new doctor. In my experience, many people that I've asked about this form reply to the effect of, "There's no one you will need to communicate with."

I think there is a common misconception among patients that adding a contact person means the clinic will want to call the contact person right away to discuss your medical care. This is certainly not the case.

Simply put, if you want anyone (family, friends, healthcare partners, other doctors) to be able to communicate with your doctor, gather medical records, call in a prescription refill request, or even just confirm appointment times, you must sign the form your doctor or hospital will provide for this purpose. On this form, list the names of *all* the people you're allowing to communicate on your behalf.

You can make changes to the form at any time. At your next doctor visit, be sure to update this vital consent-to-communicate form to ensure that your HCP, at the very least, is included on your communication consent list.

Advance Healthcare Directive

This kind of document is more involved than the previous one and generally takes one of two forms: a living will (which conveys your preferences for "extreme measures" of treatment) or a durable power of attorney (which identifies who has the legal power to make decisions about your health when you are unable to). Both require a little legwork to set up. While this can seem like a hassle, having an advance healthcare directive in place is of key importance to each and every one of us.

Here's why: if you don't prepare these documents and you become seriously ill or incapacitated, the laws in your state—rather than your wishes or those of your closest family members—may determine your care.

None of us knows when we will become unable to communicate our healthcare wishes. Elderly patients, of course, are more likely to experience symptoms that will require someone else to make healthcare choices for them. But any unforeseen accident, regardless of age or general health, can necessitate this for anyone.

Just as many of us don't plan early enough to save money for retirement, most of us don't prepare healthcare directives. It's not pleasant, but completing the forms will help those around you who may not know or remember your specific choices regarding a serious health issue.

Since it's important that your loved ones know your wishes and whom you've designated to make difficult decisions for you, it's almost imperative you have these documents prepared. Plus, you'll feel better knowing, regardless of your age, that your family members won't be burdened by having to figure this stuff out without your input.

The great news is that you can prepare these documents yourself. You don't necessarily need an attorney, but consulting one may be a source of good advice for your particular situation. That's up to you.

That said, several good websites offer a complete preparation package at a reasonable price, often less than $100, so do your due diligence. You might want to check out LegalZoom. com, which has an excellent reputation for do-it-yourself documents, and AARP, which also offers information and free downloads for forms on its site. You can research many additional options online. Just remember that, in most cases, you don't need a complex, fifty-page document prepared. Simpler is often better, according to the doctors and social workers I've asked.

In part 2, you've learned the many benefits of preparing in advance for your appointment, including how to head off potential problems, and setting yourself up for a lifetime of healthcare-navigation success. Next up, in part 3, you'll learn how to maximize your care during your appointments, treatment, and procedures, including what to expect when you're actually at the doctor's office, and money-saving tips that can drastically reduce what you pay for your prescriptions.

Part III

Maximize Your Care

INTRODUCTION TO PART III

Get the Best Out of Your Care

Having the right healthcare tools and knowing how to get started are vitally important steps on your healthcare journey. But how can you best take what you've learned so far and put it into practice when you're finally face to face with your doctor or other medical professionals?

Since maximizing our care requires us to proactively manage our own healthcare experience, it's crucial that we understand what to expect when we're actually receiving medical attention and treatment.

Knowing what to expect at your appointment frees you from some of the stress of uncertainty. This way, you'll be more relaxed in the waiting room and can focus on managing your appointment—using the plan you've already outlined on your AS form.

This marks a dramatic difference from the patient who rushes into the clinic unable to recall the name of the doctor he or she is seeing. That patient, unfortunately, is simply going to let the system take the director role.

Here in part 3, I'll get you up to speed on what's going to happen at the clinic. We'll cover what to expect when you arrive for your medical appointment, in the exam room, or at the hospital. I'll also share invaluable tips and techniques on consistently getting the best out of your care and the people who provide it.

We'll tackle questions such as the following:

- How and when should you arrive for your appointment?

- What's your objective once you're in the exam room?

- What's the best way to talk with your doctor and be heard?

- How can you convince the doctor that you need to know the other treatment options available to you?

- After your face-to-face time with the doctor, what's the follow-up plan, and why is it important to follow up?

- When you need immediate assistance with a health issue, how do you decide between going to the ER or urgent care?

- Is there a way to cut out-of-pocket expenses on prescription medications?

I'll help you answer all of these and more. Once you know what to expect when you're actually at the health clinic, you'll be able to better track and manage your own care, leading to better healthcare outcomes. Ready to begin?

Chapter 11

Arriving for
Your Appointment

Start Your Appointment Right

On the day of an appointment, many people simply arrive at the clinic at the time they were told they'd be seen, sign their name on the patient arrivals list, and wait for their name to be called. In fact, you may be asking yourself at this point why there's a whole chapter in this book dedicated to your appointment arrival.

What you might not realize is that your arrival and the check-in process play a crucial role in determining the quality of the experience you'll have—both at your current appointment and as you continue to manage any ongoing care or treatment resulting from the appointment.

Just like eating a balanced breakfast sets us up for a productive and positive day, ensuring a good beginning to your appointment sets you up for optimal healthcare success.

First impressions are important, and this is no different at the doctor's office. You want to start on the right foot, and a friendly, upbeat hello and smile will go a long way toward ensuring you communicate effectively with the doctor and the staff and get the information and treatment you need when you need it. You can call it karma or whatever you want, but an appointment that starts off positively is much more likely to continue on the same path. Conversely, I've seen time and time again how a bad attitude can negatively impact a patient's experience, throwing unnecessary frustration, wasted time, and other obstacles into his or her path.

In this chapter, I'll debunk some common misconceptions about your appointment arrival and check-in process and share valuable tips to help you optimize your healthcare experience from the moment you walk in the clinic door.

Time It Right

The first thing that factors into the success of your appointment is timing. In previous chapters, we've already covered the importance of anticipating that your appointment or procedure will take longer than expected. This mindset will help to avoid snarling your schedule for the day.

Similarly, you'll want to make sure you have enough time *before* your appointment to ensure things run smoothly at the clinic. As a good rule of thumb, always try to arrive at the check-in desk at least fifteen minutes before your scheduled appointment time. If this is your first visit with this doctor or facility, plan to arrive thirty minutes early. This allows sufficient time for most unforeseen events and any necessary check-in activities, including:

- Traffic

- Weather

- Having to stop for gas

- Parking problems

- A long line at check-in

- Paperwork that needs filling out

- Updating your contact or insurance information

Even if you plan accordingly, unexpected circumstances arise from time to time that can make you late to your doctor's appointment. Of course, the best way to minimize any potential problems resulting from running late is to communicate with the doctor's office as soon as possible.

Rather than just showing up after your scheduled appointment time, call ahead and let the office staff know you're running late. This helps the staff to streamline their team's time management by allowing them to:

- Move ahead with other patients rather than holding things up and getting everyone else behind schedule, which helps you get seen sooner, too

- Keep the doctor in the loop about last-minute schedule changes so he or she can plan accordingly

- Hold off on readying any equipment to be used for testing during your appointment until it's actually needed

When in doubt, always call the office before your appointment and ask about the arrival policy. Even though they're busy, the staff will likely appreciate your consideration, which means you'll already be starting off on the right foot.

Update Your Information

We've covered this a little in previous chapters, but it's worth mentioning again here. It's standard procedure in most offices for the receptionist to ask you, during check-in, if any of your information has changed. Most people are quick to chime in that "nothing is new," but before you say so, stop and make sure this is really true.

Consider if any of the following pieces of crucial information may have changed since the last time you were here:

- New insurance card
- New group number on your insurance
- New primary care provider
- New co-pay amount on your plan
- Change in contact phone or email

- New address
- Change in emergency contact information

The quality of your healthcare experience is heavily dependent on you providing the doctor's office with up-to-date information. For instance, your appointment confirmation won't reach you if you haven't updated your phone number. Or a billing issue could result if you don't update any changes to your insurance.

Remember, it's much easier to *prevent* a billing problem than to *correct* one. Something as simple as taking a minute to make sure the clinic has all of your current information can save you an immense amount of time and money—not to mention major frustration.

Pay Your Co-pay Now, Not Later

Not much in our healthcare journey is more complicated than understanding what our insurance will and won't pay for. One thing most of us can count on, however, is having a co-insurance payment or a co-pay due for nearly any medical appointment. The check-in desk will almost always tell you the amount up front.

A useful tip: pay that amount today.

An office visit co-pay at your doctor's clinic is typically less than $50. As a patient and a consumer, I know *I* don't want to spend time later on writing checks for something I can take care of now while I'm waiting for my appointment.

If you're charged a co-pay but believe one isn't due, I understand your hesitancy to pay now. But if it turns out you did overpay or made a payment you don't owe, it's always in the best interest of your doctor's office to return your payment. Based on my ten years of experience, patients typically do owe the co-pay, because the clinic insurance team has confirmed this ahead of time. So save yourself some time, and know that it's almost always easier on your end to take care of the co-pay at the time of your appointment.

Chapter 12

In the Exam Room

Back in the Exam Room

After you're checked in and have waited to hear your name called, your appointment is now well underway. Hopefully, you remembered to put yourself in the right frame of mind, starting with the moment you walked into the exam room.

Having the right mindset in the exam room is important, because a good attitude is one of your best tools to getting a successful healthcare experience.

This is show time. Again, you'll want to start off on the right foot, exchanging a pleasant and upbeat hello with the clinic staff member who takes you to the exam room. The nursing staff will take notice and will be ready to follow your positive lead. Once you're seated, take a deep breath and clear your mind for a moment. This will allow you to approach your upcoming chat with the doctor with a clearer head.

This is also a great time to glance over your completed AS form to remind yourself of what you'll be speaking to the doctor about and to prepare yourself to take a proactive role in your own care during the exam.

Conversely, if you spend this time complaining to the staff about your day or the long wait, or if you come off as being pressed for time, rude, or unpleasant, the negative impression this leaves can lead the staff member who is assisting you to rush through tasks. Ideally, you want the MA, nurse, NP, PA, or doctor to linger a bit longer with you in the exam room. A pleasant, prepared attitude will often achieve that goal, whereas having a negative attitude will accomplish the exact opposite and get one or more of these folks thinking, "I can't wait to get out of this room."

In this chapter, I'll cover what to expect from the moment you enter the exam room and how to approach your interactions before and during the exam with each person that you'll speak to about your health issues. When you understand what's at work, you can go in with the positive, confident attitude you need to get the best possible outcome.

Your Initial Assessment

The first person you talk to in the exam room will most likely be your doctor's nurse or MA. As we learned in part 1, the MA's job is take down some basic information from you to determine the reason for your visit, any symptoms or other discomfort you may be experiencing, and any changes to your medications or health history since the last time you were seen. The MA will also test your vitals.

All information gathered from this portion of your appointment will then be handed off to the doctor so that, even before entering the room, he or she can be prepped on how best to treat you. For this reason, it's important to thoroughly answer any questions you're asked.

Note that if you have more than one issue you'd like to be seen for, the time with the nurse or MA is your opportunity to bring these issues up. For instance, you may be primarily wanting to get the doctor's opinion about a lingering cough, but you've also been having a persistent, radiating pain in your left wrist. Be sure to speak up, but also keep in mind that your appointment may offer too limited a time to adequately address multiple issues. At that point, it's up to the nurse or MA to decide if you need another appointment to discuss any additional concerns with the doctor, or if the new complaint you brought up just became today's bigger medical issue.

If you're a new patient, have your medication list ready during your intake with the MA or nurse, and be prepared to discuss your health history. Having your HCP with you for this is ideal, but, at the very least, make sure you have these things written down. That way you'll feel confident you're providing a complete history.

In order to treat you effectively and safely, it's imperative for your new doctor to have all the big bullet points.

Once your information has been entered into the system, the staff member assisting you will let you know that the doctor will see you soon.

When the Doctor Enters

You're in the room, and there's a knock at the door. The doctor has finally arrived.

If you're like most people, you might feel a slight rush of adrenaline or anxiety at this point. This is a critical moment. Below are some tips to get the most out of your face-to-face time with your doctor.

Be Pleasant and Polite

All doctors swear an oath to treat anyone and everyone who needs their help, giving the same intense effort, aid, and succor to each and every patient. They take this oath *very* seriously; this is the foundation of why many doctors go into medicine in the first place. Even so, doctors, like the rest of us, are only human. This means, when given the choice, they prefer to interact with people who are courteous and friendly rather than those who are rude or overly aggressive.

In a nutshell, your doctor's perception of you directly affects how comfortable he or she feels with you, as well as how much time he or she's willing to talk to you during your appointment. And both of these factors impact the quality of care you will receive. If, on past visits, you've been an attentive patient and a good historian, have asked a few good questions, and were generally pleasant to interact with, then great! Chances are your doctor is immediately at ease with you upon seeing your familiar, friendly face.

If your previous appointment was in any way contentious or argumentative, or if you demanded an unrealistic amount of time, the doctor may enter the room in a more resigned or defensive mind-set. Remember, you have a right to and shouldn't settle for less than excellent healthcare and customer service. But this must be paired with a realistic expectation of each doctor visit that includes, at the very least, common courtesy. Your doctor-patient relationship is based on *several* appointments over time, after all—not just one. You want to be an "oh, yes!" patient, not an "oh, no!" one.

If you're a new patient, you have the opportunity to create that important first impression right now. Your healthcare is way too important to allow any part of the process to work against you.

Follow Your Doctor's Lead

You'll know fairly quickly if your doctor seems rushed or relaxed. Does he or she make eye contact with you and shake your hand? Does the doctor immediately say, "Hi, what brings you in today?" Or do you hear, "Wow, it's a busy day. I need to take a moment to breathe. How are you?" Your HCP may be there, too, so introduce him or her right off the bat.

If the doctor is rushed, you know you'll have to get down to healthcare business quickly. If, on the other hand, he or she takes the time to look at you and ask how you're doing, you can take a softer approach and ask *the doctor* how he or she is doing. A simple act of consideration, even one this small, can be enough to convince your doctor to spend a few more minutes with you. And the doctor will remember you for it.

Hopefully, after a bit of friendly talk, you mention the reason you're there: a pain in your knee. The doctor examines you and asks a few questions. He or she may be confident as to the cause of your pain or may want to run some further tests to narrow down or rule out possible diagnoses.

An X-ray or some lab work will confirm the doctor's initial diagnosis or suggest another one. The two of you will make a plan to follow up with another appointment in, say, two weeks. In the meantime, you will get a prescription for some medicine to reduce inflammation and help with pain. The doctor mentions the possibility of physical therapy. Or you may be referred to an orthopedic doctor, depending on the final diagnosis.

Respect the Doctor's Time

Be realistic about your expectations so you can make the most of the face-to-face time with your doctor. On average, that's going to be just a few (generally between five to eight) minutes per appointment, or a little longer if you're there for your annual wellness check. Most people—doctors, staff, and patients alike—agree that this is less than ideal, but the reality is that, given the doctor's patient load, this is all the time available for a single appointment.

Listen and Repeat What Your Doctor Says

One of the most important things you can do to get the most out of this time with your doctor is, after listening carefully to what he or she says, to repeat that information out loud to make sure you're on the same page about your diagnosis, treatment plan, and prognosis for recovery.

When your doctor is done telling you the game plan for your care, summarize what was said and repeat it out loud. Verify that you understand what you've been told and that you have all the big bullet points of advice, instructions, or other important information written down (the blank back side of your AS form is the perfect place for notes). And remember to ask the all-important question: "Are there other treatment options available to me?"

Building on our example from above, your summary might look something like this:

- Thank you, doctor. Let me take a moment to repeat this with you, okay?

- You think my arm pain is caused by a muscle sprain.

- We're going to get an X-ray of my arm.

- You want me to get some blood work done at the lab.

- You're prescribing medication. What's it called again? How often will I take it? Does this medication have any side effects, or will it interact with my current medications?

- Depending on the test results, you may:
  - Recommend physical therapy, or
  - Refer me to an orthopedic doctor.

- I should schedule a follow-up with you in two weeks.

- What's the long-term prognosis for this pain? Can I expect it to go away after treatment? Or is it likely to return?

- What other treatment options are available to me?

- Is there anything else I should be doing?

This is excellent. You listened, repeated the plan back to the doctor, and received confirmation that your summary was complete. Now you're ready to proceed with the treatment plan—confidently and completely informed.

Concluding Your Appointment

After you and the doctor have gone over your issue, formulated the next step, and determined whether a follow-up visit is needed, your doctor may offer you a printed summary of the plan so you have it in writing. Alternately, after a surgery, an ER visit, or a hospital stay, you'll get discharge instructions.

In either case, fantastic! This is useful because it will likely include your treatment plan and your updated medication list. If you're taking a truly proactive approach to your healthcare and keeping a file or binder for your health history, that's where this paperwork should be kept.

However, even if you get this kind of printout from the clinic, you cannot rely on it alone. It's possible that much of the information from your doctor visit is not fully updated on the printout, and it may detail only *part* of the full treatment plan picture.

This is where your AS form becomes an invaluable resource for every doctor's appointment you have. A completed AS form, paired with your doctor's after-visit summary, gives you a much more complete overview of all the information you may need to refer back to weeks, months, or even years later.

Remember, you are always your most valuable healthcare advocate!

Chapter 13

The Emergency Room
or Urgent Care?

A Rude Awakening

I still remember the shock of waking from a sound sleep to intense pain and pressure coming from my left flank.

It was half past three in the morning when I shot straight up in bed. The pain was so severe that my hand flew to my side, half expecting to find an open wound. There was none, but still I flailed and winced. Thankfully, my wife was there to rush me to the ER.

By the time we arrived, I was nearly incoherent with the pain. The check-in staff saw me and nodded knowingly. "Looks like you're passing a kidney stone," one offered. I was roomed immediately, and after a few injections of a strong medication, I felt the intense relief of that relentless pain subsiding. A blood draw, a CT scan, and an X-ray later, the diagnosis was complete.

This stone-passing incident, the first of several I would experience, led to a three-hour ER stay—which came with what was, at the time, a surprisingly expensive price tag.

As serious as my symptoms were, it turned out the cause of my pain was far from life-threatening. I've since learned that you can easily be treated for a kidney-stone episode at an urgent care center, which is how I've chosen to seek treatment for recurring instances of this painful condition. There was no way, however, you could have convinced me I needed to go anywhere but the ER in the midst of such a frightening and unfamiliar experience that first night.

Perfect Storm of Confusing Choices

Each year in the United States, more than 130 million patients visit the ER. On average, that's more than 40 percent of all US citizens. With that kind of traffic, you'd think we'd all be experts on ER visits by now. But you'd be wrong.

Sadly, the ER remains one of the most misunderstood resources in the healthcare industry. If and when we should go to the ER, and what we can expect once we get there, remain some of the most perplexing and stressful health-related questions most of us will ever face. And worse, if we don't take the time to learn this information ahead of time—and all too few of us do—we'll be faced with these same questions in the worst moments of our lives: when we or our loved ones are seriously injured or ill.

Since our lives and those of our loved ones can *literally* depend on decisions such as if or when to go to the ER, it's of dire importance to educate ourselves about this topic.

And since ER visits also come with an inevitably hefty price tag, it's important that we understand what other options are available and how to decide which one is the better option for us in any given situation.

It's important to note there are times you *absolutely* need to go to your local ER if your illness warrants that level of immediate care. In these cases, if you wait until the ER visit is less of an inconvenience for you or your family, you risk an even more serious illness. Doctors always preach that early detection and treatment are keys to healthcare success. Even a young patient who accidently ingests too many pain relievers can risk permanent internal organ damage if he or she is not treated within a very short period of time.

The ER nursing staff and most doctors won't tell you that your ER stay wasn't necessary or that you could have been seen by your primary care doctor or at an urgent care center instead. They will speak among themselves about it, but not to you. That's not their job. For this reason, taking the time to become educated about this topic can improve the type of care you receive, the timeliness of the treatment, and, most certainly, the cost. As a patient, it's always in your best interest to know ahead of time which service option is best for you.

In this chapter, you'll learn when to go to the ER and what to expect there, so you'll be able to make informed decisions while under stress in a potential health crisis. We'll also explore an increasingly popular alternative to the ER for serious health concerns that aren't life- or limb-threatening: urgent care centers.

The ER and Urgent Care: A Side-by-Side Comparison

Trying to decide whether urgent care or the ER is more appropriate can be tricky, but there's one rule of thumb you can keep in mind to help guide your decision-making: urgent care is generally an excellent choice for conditions and injuries that are not life- or limb-threatening.

Urgent care facilities are much more state-of-the art than in years past. They're staffed by physicians and a skilled medical team, and some have X-ray equipment, a lab, or both. These facilities can address a variety of serious health concerns.

I've assembled the table below to give you a better sense of what kinds of conditions merit a trip to your local urgent care center or, conversely, the ER.

When to go to the emergency room	When urgent care may be appropriate
Heart attack symptoms such as chest pain, jaw pain, left arm pain	Minor pain, abdominal or back pain
Stroke symptoms (FAST):	Vomiting, diarrhea, dehydration
• F: facial drooping • A: arm weakness • S: speech difficulties • T: time	Fevers, flu, cough
	Sore throat, strep throat, sinus infection
Severe sudden headache	Rash or skin issues, pinkeye, insect or animal bites
Nonresponsive or unconscious	Common cuts and lacerations
Difficulty breathing, shortness of breath, or choking	Urination discomfort, urinary tract infections
Significant broken bones or uncontrolled bleeding from lacerations	Minor burns
	Sprains or small broken bones
Moderate to severe burns	Most sports injuries
Drug overdoses or ingestion of poisons	Asthma flare-ups
Severe bleeding	Follow-up care after a PCP or ER visit (i.e., removing stitches or checking on a wound) X-rays and lab testing
Neck and spinal injuries	
Infant fevers	You know what your illness is, but can't get a same-day appointment with your primary care doctor
Seizures	
Severe abdominal pain	
Serious eye injuries, loss of vision	
Possible need for surgery	
Your gut telling you the symptom/injury is life-threatening	

While a trip to urgent care is generally more wallet-friendly than an ER visit, comparing the benefits of the ER and urgent care centers is never simply a matter of cost effectiveness. The much larger issue at play is which option will offer the most appropriate medical care for your current health problem in the most appropriate time frame.

It's not widely known, but there's a history of ER overuse among a limited number of patients. Some, for instance, checked into our ER more than twice every week, often for issues that could have been adequately addressed at their regular doctor's office or urgent care. There are also instances of patients utilizing the ER for coughs and colds when their primary care physician (PCP) could have easily treated such illnesses. This practice does much harm to easily overburdened ER facilities, causing patient wait times to skyrocket. Worse, it also stretches the hospital's resources even thinner, since hospitals typically collect far less than they bill for their services.

Estimates vary widely, but one reliable study showed that nearly half of the patients who visited an ER were there because their PCP's office was closed. Wow! Other doctor surveys estimate that up to 27 percent of ER visits are nonurgent. As a result, insurance companies have substantially hiked ER patient out-of-pocket co-pays as a financial disincentive. ERs are doing their part by working to assign patients to PCPs. That way, patients feel they have someone to contact before going to the ER, especially in clearly nonurgent cases. And most PCPs offer someone on call after hours to speak to and assist patients.

What to Expect at the ER

In addition to the substantial cost, a long wait time at the ER is typically one of the biggest challenges you'll face once you get checked in at the front desk. Multiple factors influence these long wait times, but there are two main reasons that you should be aware of.

First, due to the realities of our healthcare system, hospitals all over the country face a shortage of adequate doctors, staff, and space to see and treat as many patients as they see come through their doors. And second, due to the very serious nature of the health issues many ER patients are seen for, the order in which all patients are seen and treated is managed by a triage system. This system exists with the sole purpose of saving lives.

As an ER patient, you will be triaged by an experienced RN who provides an experienced initial assessment and assigns an acuity level (usually a number from one to five) as to how serious your medical issue is. That information is relayed to the ER charge nurse and to the physicians and their team. Chest pain patients are typically immediately placed in a room, while patients with abdominal pain (the most common ER condition) are likely to get a lower acuity rating.

In addition to chest pains, patients with the following types of conditions are typically prioritized for immediate attention:

- Possible stroke symptoms

- Serious bleeding

- Drug overdoses

- Serious injuries from auto- or work-related accidents

- Trauma

- Nonresponsiveness

If you're there for most other conditions, expect your ER wait time to be significant, as reflected by your acuity assignment. The ER's clinical staff is efficient, talented, and able to handle a difficult workload, and they are happiest when your treatment works and they can send you home feeling better. Truly, if you've never seen them in action before, it's amazing to watch an ER trauma team deliver care to a critically ill patient.

Patients without insurance or those covered by state Medicaid programs often utilize the ER because they know they'll be seen regardless of their ability to pay. No patient should ever be left behind.

On that note, it's also worth mentioning that, though the ER where I worked might not accept your insurance coverage, we were strictly forbidden from mentioning that to a patient at check-in. The hospital simply did not want a seriously ill patient to leave until he or she received treatment. That's a good health policy, but it can be a potentially devastating financial issue for the patient. The possibility of your local ER having a similar policy is something to be aware of. When in doubt, always ask!

What to Expect at Urgent Care

As previously mentioned, urgent care facilities are ideal for non-life-threatening conditions—that persistent stomach issue or the cut that needs stitches. Even a broken finger or toe are easily handled by an urgent care facility.

At urgent care, you'll likely be seen and treated considerably more quickly than at an ER. Indeed, one of the biggest complaints from people in the ER is the length of wait time. Even after you're finally placed in an exam room, your wait can be several more hours before you're discharged. Urgent care facilities are often well staffed, and, because most patients are not seriously ill, they are able to treat patients and send them home more quickly.

Urgent care facilities will also be very up front with you as to the cost of any services and whether they accept your health insurance or not. They are commonly for-profit centers, which means that if they aren't certain your insurance will cover your treatment, they may ask you to pay in advance and request reimbursement from your insurance provider. It's worth noting that this can be an arduous and time-consuming process, so be sure to educate yourself about your insurance plan's options for urgent care.

In fact, your insurance provider is likely to offer you an incentive to visit urgent care facilities over the ER when your current medical issue can be safely and adequately addressed in this way. For instance, you might be offered a significantly reduced co-pay compared to the ER. (I've seen patients pay $50 urgent care co-pays versus $100 to $300 ER co-pays, since co-pays are typically due regardless of the medical issue you're facing.) Additionally, some insurance providers pay a larger percentage of your urgent care visits compared to the ER.

That said, be sure to check—before you head to urgent care—that the facility you've selected accepts your insurance. This is especially important if you have an HMO or one of the many new hybrid plans that insurance providers are offering. In these cases, the ER—by law or by choice—is sometimes more likely to accept your insurance, including state Medicaid programs. For better or worse, the ER will almost always see every patient, even if your insurance isn't accepted by them—but you may be surprised to be sent a big bill as a result.

Before and After Your ER or Urgent Care Visit

It's up to you to decide whether the ER or urgent care (or even a drop-in clinic at your local pharmacy) best matches your immediate health concern. Since you never know when a sudden or severe illness or injury might strike, it's often difficult to prepare in advance for such a trip. However, there is one thing you can do to make sure you're prepared ahead of time, and this is something that an alarming number of people never do.

Take the time to educate yourself about which facilities—both ERs and urgent care centers—in your area accept your insurance and what kind of co-pay or other expenses you can expect to incur if the need for such a visit arises. To do this, call your insurance provider and discuss your options for ER and urgent care visits *when you're well*—the sooner the better, if you haven't done this yet.

Once you've done this, you can rest easier, knowing that if and when a sudden, serious health issue *does* come up, you'll know exactly where to go for help in a hurry. This will help you avoid adding untold unnecessary stress and anxiety to the existing strain of dealing with a sudden health issue or crisis. I recall many cases where the patient or family member told the ambulance team the exact hospital they needed to go to. If the medical situation is not a minute-to-minute, life-threatening one, the ambulance team can often accommodate the request.

Before you leave the ER or urgent care, it's always a great idea to ask for a printed summary of your visit for your own records. You should also share this document with your PCP. (Your doctor can request your medical records from the ER or urgent care if more information is needed.) Remember to mention any ER or urgent care visits to your doctor and the nursing staff at your next appointment. You'll almost always be instructed by the ER or urgent care team to follow up with your doctor within a few days.

If your ER visit was serious, call your PCP in a timely manner in case the doctor decides this issue merits you coming in for a follow-up appointment.

Chapter 14

At the Hospital

When my wife, Mary, was in the hospital numerous times during her battle with breast cancer, we both focused on one thing: going home. This said, thank goodness for hospitals and the staff there. They are generally incredibly compassionate and wonderful people, and they do amazing things for patients and the patient's family. Even the food is a little better these days. But what drove us—and what should motivate you—is to get well enough to *leave* the hospital.

It's estimated that the average hospital stay costs upwards of $5,000 per day—and that's just for the basics. Everyone is motivated to get you home and out of the hospital: the hospital staff, the doctor, your insurance company, your family, and especially you. The steps you take to understand the treatment plan and to work toward your goal of going home will help you reach the point when you are discharged.

Since streamlining the length of time you spend in the hospital means moving forward with testing, recovery, and the overall plan to get you home, it's vital that you know what to expect at the hospital and how to communicate with (and, at times, even *direct*) the staff.

It's important to understand that you are one of probably hundreds of patients at your hospital. There are thousands of moving parts (medical staff, machines, tests, surgeries, medications, etc.), and you're the reason for all of it during your hospital stay. As I'll discuss in more detail later, getting everyone and everything at the hospital on the same page is difficult at best. But we have to start somewhere.

The last thing you want is to simply drift through this system rather than steer your own course. Knowing what to expect at the hospital will keep you focused on healing faster. It will also help you to picture being home again and returning to your regular life, work, and family, helping you to maintain an optimistic and happy outlook—crucial components of a successful recovery. When you have realistic expectations about potential challenges, then even if you have some setbacks during your stay, you can remain focused on your goal of getting better.

If you don't know what's happening next, where you stand in your recovery, or if you're just waiting for the next nurse to bring a pill or hoping someone will have some news, you're more likely to languish. After all, how can you work toward a goal if you don't know what that goal is? Just as you manage an efficient doctor's appointment by asking questions, repeating back the treatment plan, and having the medical staff keep you regularly updated on your progress, you and your HCP should adopt a similarly proactive attitude in order to successfully navigate a hospital stay.

In this chapter, I'll share how to navigate and stream-line your hospital stay by managing your expectations and understanding how best to communicate with the hospital staff, including your doctors. Armed with what you'll learn here, you and your HCP will be able to keep your recovery moving in the right direction, working together with the team of doctors, nurses, and MAs to make sure they know how best to help you reach your goal of being well enough to go home.

What to Expect at the Hospital

Many of the same strategies we utilize for a doctor's office appointment are applicable when you're admitted to the hos-pital. There are, of course, some differences.

For starters, your hospital care is often managed by a medical support team made up of nurses, an MA, and your doctor (and, if you're at a teaching hospital, your doctor's PA and residents). I liken a hospital to a large ship. It's not very nimble, and it takes a long time to get it moving and a tremendous effort to keep it moving forward.

Hospitals have many moving parts, and it's quite possi-ble that each functions with varying levels of efficiency. I'm not sure that will ever change. Still, the comfort of knowing you're on that "big ship" can be very reassuring, especially when you're seriously ill.

Let's look at the key role players at the hospital and how they work with you.

- *Registration and admitting staff:* These are important staffers who confirm your insurance and demographic data and prepare your chart for the medical team.

- *MAs:* The workhorse team members, these folks assist the entire medical floor staff. The medical assistant may be the person you're in contact with most during your stay.

- *Nursing staff:* They will administer your medications, verify your vitals, explain the treatment plan, and answer medical questions when the doctor isn't there. They also regularly update your medical chart and communicate directly with the doctor and will be with the doctor when he or she sees you.

- *PAs and NPs:* As mentioned earlier, a physician assistant or nurse practitioner might fill in for a doctor to provide updates to you. Both are trained to administer treatment and can perform in-room procedures. They are approachable and will typically spend time answering your questions.

- *Residents and medical students:* At teaching hospitals, these students (many are actually doctors by definition) travel with the doctor assigned to you. They also might check in with you on their own during the day. They have less training and experience, but can still be a great resource for getting your questions answered.

- *Technicians for tests and procedures:* If you're in the hospital, chances are you're going to have tests and lab work completed, so you'll likely see these staffers regularly.

- *Social workers:* These valuable and often underutilized health team members can help you and your family by providing more complete and less rushed explanations of your diagnoses and treatment plan. They will take the time to make sure you understand and are key resources for communicating with your HCP and your family. They can also help you arrange for after-hospital care or rehabilitation services.

- *Doctors:* It doesn't matter if you're in a clinic, surgery center, or hospital, it's always show time when your doctor sees you. In the few minutes the doctor is with you, you'll find out more about your diagnosis and treatment than at any other time.

Get the Most from Your Time with the Doctor

A hospital stay is as much a waiting game as it is anything else, and knowing when the doctor is coming to see you can be a real mystery. Doctors are busy—we know that. They have a limited amount of time for each patient. And we know nothing replaces face-to-face time with your doctor. So taking advantage of the daily—or twice daily—meeting is critical to you receiving good, timely care.

For the best results, you need to be especially alert and focused for your all-important daily medical "briefing" with the doctor. For each of these meetings, you, the patient, have three primary objectives:

- **Review your condition with the doctor.** Again, why are you here at the hospital? Yes, this is all too obvious . . . to you. But you may be seeing a completely different doctor during the next round of doctor visits since doctors' schedules vary. For instance, if you're in the cardiac unit, your regular doctor may be off for the weekend. The new doctor has looked at your chart and knows the basics, but you may need to fill in some of the blanks.

- **Update the doctor on your condition.** How are you feeling today versus yesterday? Is anything new or different, better or worse, since the day before? You may be taking medication for your condition. If so, how is that working? Are you experiencing any side effects?

- **Discuss the treatment plan and the date you get to leave the hospital.** Now's the time to see what the plan is going forward. Are there more tests planned? Is the doctor pleased with your progress, and, if so, when are you going home? The estimate of when you get to leave varies day to day, doctor to doctor, so if you were told something different yesterday, remind your doctor of that. Remember: the plan is to get you better and out of the hospital. Knowing the specifics of the plan to achieve this will motivate you to do your part to get well enough to go home.

Doctor visits usually occur in the morning, but their timing tends to be up in the air, depending on a variety of factors. Ask your nurse when he or she thinks the doctor will see you. Say that you want your HCP with you to document what the doctor says. Just as with a regular doctor's office appointment, the doctor's briefing at the hospital is too important an event to rely on yourself alone to remember everything that is discussed.

Your nurse will also most likely be in the room when the doctor and the team are present and can help summarize and repeat the treatment plan if your HCP isn't available. (You can even ask the nurse to take notes for you if your

HCP can't be there.) Refer to your notes from the doctor's briefing during the rest of the day to stay motivated and keep your eyes on the prize: getting well so you can go home!

Stay on Top of Shift Changes

One crucial reality to be aware of is that, every eight to twelve hours, your nurse, MA, and the entire support team on your floor clock out and go home, and other staff who work the same jobs come in and take their places. After all, the hospital stays open for business twenty-four hours a day, seven days a week, every single day of the year.

Just before a shift change, a meeting takes place where patients are handed off to the next shift. A discussion of the patient's medical condition and treatment plan occurs during this meeting, but it's possible that some pieces of information may be left out or misunderstood, or that the pace of things may slow down a bit while the new shift is getting up to speed. Confusion or delays that result from this can be frustrating from the patient's point of view, but no one is making things more difficult intentionally. Rather, shift changes are simply a natural reality of how things work at the hospital.

For example, you may know the doctor mentioned you would be getting up out of bed after a surgery to do a walk around the floor, and then a shift change kicks in. The doctor mentioned your upcoming walk hours earlier, but no one comes to help you out of bed and around the floor. That's when it's time to speak up and remind or inform your new shift nurse that you're supposed to be out of bed.

To be fair, most nurses are amazing, and the MAs and even the front-desk staff are typically very hardworking and have your best care in mind. Still, shift changes can result in a change in the continuity of care you're provided—for better, worse, or sometimes just different. In fact, it's possible the shift change will result in you having a nursing staff that may push your diagnosis, procedure, and treatment program even more assertively, so it may be a positive situation when a shift change occurs.

Even so, whenever the new nursing staff stopped into my wife's room to write their names on the whiteboard at a shift change, as an HCP I sometimes felt the air go out of my sails. That's because shift changes can lead to a sense of confusion about who knows what and/or a loss of momentum that was building with the previous nursing team. This is a major complaint among patients in the hospital and their loved ones, so it's something to be aware of so you can successfully navigate this shift in the tides.

To avoid negative continuity changes, be sure to write down somewhere permanent everything your medical support team writes on your whiteboard (or ideally, have your HCP write it down). That way, you have everything in one place even after the old information gets erased. Also, ask your RN or MA to write your wellness plan down so you know your schedule for the day or next few days.

Put this list on the wall or at the head of your bed. Look at it frequently, and ask questions about when events such as testing are going to take place. Even just seeing the list may spur the RN or other staff to action.

Having this list posted will give you a general picture of what to expect today, tomorrow, and maybe even the next few days. Remember: your only job while you're in the hospital is to get well enough to go home. When you understand what's happening every day to reach that goal (and understand that this list will change), you'll be motivated to do your part as well.

Bottom line: you're *much* more likely to receive better care and go home sooner if you take this proactive approach.

Get Help from Social Workers

Hospitals and larger clinics often employ a team of social workers. This group of people is an invaluable resource to patients—but only if patients know how to best utilize this resource.

The list of services social workers might provide to a hospital patient is extensive. For instance, they can help your aging parent find a temporary nursing home or rehabilitation center while he or she recovers from an illness, injury, or surgery.

Social workers are also able to perform some of the duties your regular HCP helps with.

It's important to know that you might not be automatically assigned a social worker during your hospital stay. A doctor or the nursing staff typically needs to request one for you. But if you confidently ask for this assistance, most hospitals will provide one for you. Here are some other examples of what a social worker can do for you during your hospital stay:

- Help explain your diagnosis and treatment plan (any time another professional can help explain a complex diagnosis and treatment options, even if it's already been explained to you by someone else, you should take advantage of this offering)

- Arrange for services or medical equipment you might need after you leave the hospital

- Identify good options for nursing care or rehabilitation facilities

- Assist with mental health or grief counseling services

- Help prepare a patient's advance care directive

As with preparing to see your doctor, write down any questions for the social worker in advance. He or she will appreciate your preparation, and you'll be ready to listen and take notes to help you improve your understanding of your care.

Chapter 15

Save Money on Your Prescriptions

A Dollar Saved . . .

Nationally, we spend nearly $400 billion each year on prescription medications. That's staggering. But many Americans don't realize there are a variety of options available to help us get the medications we need without breaking the bank.

Since getting our share of the healthcare pie means cutting costs without cutting quality, anything you can do to save on prescription-drug costs is well worth the effort.

In this chapter, I'll teach you cost-saving tips to help you stay healthy and save some cash while you're at it.

Ask Your Doctor for Free Samples

One of the best ways to save money on your prescriptions is to ask your doctor for free samples of any of the medications you're taking—especially the more expensive ones. No one is sure of the exact number, but it's estimated that in 2015 more than $6 billion was spent on distribution of free pharmaceutical samples to physicians. That's a lot of free medicine up for grabs!

Drug-company representatives give doctors free samples to give to their patients to try, hoping that the patients will keep using the medication. It's a marketing effort—one that you can take advantage of to save yourself some money.

Chances are that your doctor won't have samples of all of your medications—maybe just a few, or maybe even none. It's probably not worth asking if your medication costs only a few dollars, but it's a good idea to get into the habit of asking.

The underlying truth, though, is that free samples do impact the overall cost of prescription medications, as do marketing costs and the incredibly expensive process of taking a new drug to market. You can decide for yourself how you feel about the free sample program. The samples may be free, but maybe not in a big-picture sense. However, I believe that anything that saves you money—while still providing the quality medical care you deserve and need—is of benefit to you. I get a kick out of patients who regularly—politely and without a sense of entitlement—ask for samples of their current medications. Good for them!

Other Ways to Save

- **Generic Brands:** If you're using a name-brand medication, find out if there's a generic version available, or if one is expected on the market soon.

- **Similar Medications:** You may find that the out-of-pocket cost of your prescribed medication is hundreds of dollars, even with your insurance company paying part of the cost. If so, ask your doctor if there is a similar medication that provides the same benefits but at a lower cost. The pharmacist may know of a substitute medication and can even ask your doctor about this on your behalf. Ultimately, you and your doctor should decide if this new option works for you.

- **Coupons:** The next time you visit the pharmacy, ask the technician at the counter if there are any current coupons available that will help reduce the cost of your prescriptions.

- **Prescription Drug Savings Card:** Your insurance provider or your pharmacy might offer a free savings card you can use for discounted prescription benefits.

In part 3, you've learned how to navigate your experience at the doctor's clinic, ER, urgent care center, and hospital with the confidence and knowhow you need to get the best out of the system. We've covered valuable techniques to help you save money, avoid problems with your care, and communicate effectively with everyone on your medical team. Next up, in part 4, you'll learn how to make sure all the hard work you've done so far doesn't go to waste while learning how to manage your follow-up care.

Part IV

Follow Up

INTRODUCTION TO PART IV

Stay on Top of Your Healthcare Game

By now, you're becoming an expert on how to proactively manage your healthcare journey, but there are a few final tips and tricks to learn in order to fully stay on top of your game.

You—and probably your HCP, too—have invested a tremendous amount of time and thought into your healthcare up to this point. You have prepared for your appointments by reviewing your medical condition, had your questions ready for the doctor and nursing staff, and asked for clarification of the treatment plan going forward.

Great work! You're mostly there, but the one final critical component is to follow through and follow up on that plan.

Here's why: just as you need to finish the entire bottle of antibiotics your doctor has prescribed for an infection, you need to complete—to the last letter—any other treatment plan outlined to achieve the best health results. Patients often follow a plan until they start feeling better, at which point they may be inclined to stop their treatment. I hear stories all the time from doctors or nursing staff about patients returning to the clinic with similar symptoms. "They should have continued with their physical therapy," they say, or "We prescribed medication for two weeks. Why did the patient stop taking it after just one?"

Since many treatment plans include stages of treatments, it's vital to make sure you complete the entire course of any medication, therapies, or other treatment plans outlined by your doctor for your medical condition. Keep in mind that you may also need to see your doctor after each of these stages during the course of treatment, so stay in touch with your doctor's staff about how you're doing.

Your follow-through and proactive attitude will lead to better health outcomes for you, with the added benefit of demonstrating to your doctor and the medical staff that you're committed to your healthcare success. Communicating with the doctor's staff is equally important if your results were bad *or* good. Your doctor wants to know if his or her diagnoses are correct, if the recommendations were successful, and, of course, if the results were not.

Here in part 4, we'll cover how to manage the ins and outs of your care after an appointment, procedure, or hospital stay, including topics like getting additional medical advice.

We'll tackle questions like these two:

- When should I get a second opinion?

- What can I do to help my loved ones get on board with helping manage my (and their own!) health more proactively?

Once you master these final techniques for getting the best out of the system, you'll be ready to go forth and share what you've learned with others, helping create a new paradigm shift in how the people you love manage their health. And when this happens, we all benefit.

Chapter 16

Get a Second Opinion

The Value of a Fresh Set of Eyes

A recent study by the renowned Mayo Clinic showed that nearly 90 percent of patients who sought a second opinion left that appointment with a revised or completely different diagnosis than they were first given. Read that again.

Yes. I said *90* percent.

Nine out of ten patients who sought a second opinion received medical advice that significantly altered their diagnosis. Now take a moment to think about how many patients *don't* get a second opinion and how seriously their health may be impacted by this.

Since our health is much too important to risk on a faulty or incomplete diagnosis, it's important to get a second opinion. In fact, if you're diagnosed with a serious illness or a major surgery, a second opinion may actually be required by your insurance company. Doctors are generally highly competent, and they all have in common wanting the best for their patients. That said, even doctors sometimes make mistakes or don't get enough information to get a full picture of what may be going on with your health. Or they may just have differing opinions on how to treat your illness.

Perhaps a key piece of information (a symptom, a medication interaction, etc.) may slip through the cracks, or perhaps your primary doctor simply has never seen a case like yours before and mistakes your injury or illness for something else. The old saying "two heads are better than one" definitely applies here. Getting a second opinion gives you and your healthcare team the best possible chance at successfully identifying and treating whatever medical issue you're dealing with.

In this chapter, I'll cover when to seek out a second opinion and offer tips for how to go about this. Once you get that second take on your medical issue and how best to proceed, you can rest easier that you're making a more fully informed decision about your care.

When to Get a Second Opinion

First off, it's important to retain your perspective on the situation when your doctor gives you unpleasant news, like recommending surgery. When you hear those words come out of the doctor's mouth, your fight-or-flight reflex starts to kick in. As we've learned, this is not an opportune time to make any final decisions about your health on your own. Bringing your HCP with you to your appointment is a great way to help manage this problem, since he or she is able to keep a cooler head.

Don't hesitate to tell your doctor you want to ask for a second opinion. This also gives the doctor the opportunity to take more time to explain your medical condition and the procedure or treatment plan.

Another issue that often comes up surrounding this topic is the concern among patients that you'll offend your physician if you ask for another doctor's opinion. I'm here to tell you not to worry about this. Getting a second opinion is incredibly common in the healthcare industry. Particularly when it comes to surgeries or other intensive procedures or treatments, doctors understand that you want to be absolutely sure you're choosing the right treatment plan before you proceed.

Situations when it's a good idea to get a second opinion include the following:

- Your doctor suggests a major surgery (i.e., heart, brain, major organ, cancer related, etc.)
- You've been diagnosed with a new major medical condition
- The diagnosis will have a significant impact on your long-term quality of life
- You are uncomfortable with or unsure about the diagnosis
- Your insurance company requires it

You'll also need to verify that your insurance company will pay for a second opinion. In many cases, this is covered. Medicare, for instance, may even pay for a third opinion if the first two doctors issued differing diagnoses. In any case, if you're considering getting a second opinion, call your insurance provider and discuss your options.

How to Get a Second Opinion

Once you've verified that your insurance plan will cover a second opinion, it's time to get your appointment scheduled. You're an expert at this by now, of course, but there are a few things to keep in mind when scheduling an appointment for a second opinion.

First, I recommend that you find a doctor who is not affiliated with your doctor. Select one from an entirely different practice or healthcare provider.

You also need to be specific when contacting the second-opinion doctor's office about the type of appointment you're scheduling. Doctors have specific time slots assigned for second-opinion appointments. Because of this, keep in mind that you may be waiting days or even weeks to see the doctor for this kind of appointment.

The second-opinion doctor will also need access to your medical records from your initial doctor. Once you have identified the second-opinion doctor, request the medical records yourself so you can track this process and make sure the information transfer takes place before your upcoming appointment. The last thing you want is to wait weeks for your second opinion, only to have the appointment delayed even further because someone forgot to send over your medical chart. Staying on top of the process will help avoid this problem and bring you increased peace of mind.

Finally, once you actually get your second opinion, it may be the case that you're now looking at two conflicting medical opinions. When this happens, how do you know which one is the correct one?

There are several suggested approaches to this challenge. Scheduling a follow-up appointment with your original doctor is a good start. Have your first doctor speak with the second-opinion doctor to discuss the results. This will allow both doctors a chance to share information and further discuss your case. If they reach a consensus diagnosis or treatment plan, you can then decide if their advice is acceptable to you.

Most times, when the doctors agree to work together, this is effective. If this doesn't work, however, and they continue to have differing opinions, it may be time to bring in a third doctor to research the first two opinions and come up with a separate conclusion.

Ultimately, you'll be the one deciding which treatment or surgery is best for you. This is a fantastic opportunity to speak with and gather opinions from other patients who have experienced a similar medical condition and undergone a surgery or treatment comparable to the one being recommended to you. (You can find support groups, as well as a plethora of useful information, using a simple Google search.) Having your HCP help with this process will make what can seem like an overwhelming situation much easier to manage.

Getting a second opinion takes real work, but that process fits in with our new goal of taking the extra steps necessary to become informed, confident, and better-prepared patients. Remember: better-prepared patients receive better healthcare and, consequently, achieve better health.

Chapter 18

A Healthier Tomorrow

Your Healthcare Action Plan

With all the information, tools, and techniques you've now mastered, you're prepared to navigate the healthcare maze with comfort and confidence. Now it's your turn to implement these concepts into your healthcare routine. In doing so, you'll be leaps ahead of other patients—I guarantee it. And since we know that patients will continue to have to compete for valuable face-to-face time with the doctor, that's an important advantage to have.

I also recommend incorporating your personal healthcare notes, AS forms, medication lists, insurance documents, and other helpful patient information into a single healthcare-summary notebook. Once you get yourself organized, you'll be a well-prepared patient, ready to stare down the challenge of managing your healthcare journey, and ready to do the same for others.

Once you become more proactive in your approach to managing your healthcare, you'll not only improve your health but also achieve greater peace of mind. Your family will appreciate that you're taking good care of yourself. Even better, you'll be setting a good example for them to follow.

Your Partner in Healthcare Success

I'm so very excited to have had the opportunity to share my experience and observations with you in the pages of this book! And the journey doesn't have to end here. I welcome your feedback, questions, stories, and any tips you want to share about effectively navigating the healthcare system. You can reach me by email at Dale@preppedpatients.com. I also invite you to visit my website, http://www.preppedpatients.com/, and join the growing community of prepped patients there.

On my site, you can find additional resources to help you and your loved ones stay healthy, including a downloadable copy of the AS form. The site also features a blog, videos, and news updates about the book, as well as information on where you can meet me at book signings, lectures, and more.

The community we are creating together will continue to evolve, just as medical care, treatment options, and insurance coverage continue to change over time. Together, we can work for a healthier, happier future.

A Healthier Tomorrow . . . for All of Us

First and foremost, this book is for you, the patient. I wrote it because I'm passionate about patients receiving the care they deserve and seeing improved health outcomes.

You can and should be empowered to manage your own healthcare. You *need* to be, because the system is tricky to navigate, and your health is on the line. Your healthcare partner is a valuable resource, but even the best HCP won't be able to attend all of your appointments, tests, and surgical procedures. That's why *you* are, and always will be, your own best healthcare partner and advocate.

Work proactively to ensure good healthcare outcomes for yourself in every way you can, and help those around you to learn by your good example. Share what you've learned, and keep on learning as you continue your journey. What better gift can you give to the people you care about than empowering them to live healthier, happier lives?

I often consider my place in the world. I'm sure you do the same. I feel an incredible sense of purpose and passion in helping patients better understand their own healthcare. The increased confidence that comes with understanding and knowing how to navigate the system and communicate with doctors and other medical personnel and support staff makes a world of difference in achieving better health outcomes.

Every day in my work I see the need for the knowledge I've shared with you here, and I've seen firsthand how vital these strategies and techniques are in helping patients reach their healthcare goals.

I know that together we can build a future where we and our loved ones are armed with the knowledge, confidence, and proactive mindset we need to ensure that each of us receives the best possible care and treatment for any health challenge that comes along.

The future looks bright! And the journey has only just begun . . .

ABOUT THE AUTHOR

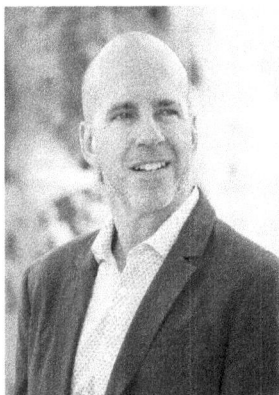

Dale White is *the* expert when it comes to navigating the complex healthcare system. He has worked in more than twenty clinics and a busy hospital at a leading university medical school. With over a decade of healthcare experience, he has provided support to more than 50,000 patients as they began their visits to emergency rooms, medical clinics, and surgery centers.

White's career in healthcare began as a volunteer in the ER when his wife was in the final stages of her thirteen-year battle with breast cancer. He left the corporate world for the more rewarding work he found helping people who are sick, scared, and unsure. His career as a healthcare worker, combined with the skills learned running a consulting company, have provided White with invaluable insights, which he now shares to help patients more confidently take control of their healthcare experiences.

White currently works in an outpatient surgery clinic. He lives in Rancho Mission Viejo, California.